RE-CYCLING

Taking up Bicycling Again as an Adult

Bruce Wynkoop

AuthorHouse™
1663 Liberty Drive
Bloomington, IN 47403
www.authorhouse.com
Phone: 1-800-839-8640

© 2009 Bruce Wynkoop. All rights reserved.

No part of this book may be reproduced, stored in a retrieval system, or transmitted by any means without the written permission of the author.

First published by AuthorHouse 7/17/2009

ISBN: 978-1-4389-9913-5 (sc)

Printed in the United States of America
Bloomington, Indiana
This book is printed on acid-free paper.

Dedication

To: My sister, Chris, and my friend, Linda, for encouraging me to finish the book and never saying, "You must be crazy!"

My good friend, Eric, who pushed me into my first week-long bike ride and with whom I have shared many great cycling moments.

My good friend, Steve, with whom I have shared many great bike trips.

To Chris —
A great sister and a great friend. Thanks for your encouragement!
Love,
Bruce

Contents

Dedication		v
Introduction		ix
Chapter 1	Getting Started	1
Chapter 2	Buying the Bike	6
Chapter 3	Starting to Ride	11
Chapter 4	Shifting	24
Chapter 5	Equipment	30
Chapter 6	Commuting	37
Chapter 7	Accidents	41
Chapter 8	More Comfortable Riding	46
Chapter 9	More Serious Riding	50
Chapter 10	Why Cyclists "Do That"	61
Chapter 11	How Motorists Can Help Cyclists	65
Chapter 12	The Love of Cycling	71

Introduction

In 1976 I was a young police officer in St. Paul, Minnesota. I had been an athlete my entire life, still played many sports, and was in reasonably good shape. One night my partner and I answered a call for a petty theft in progress at a local convenience store. We went to the store and encountered two suspects who were accused by the owner of trying to steal a small amount of candy and handled the call accordingly, telling the suspects to step out to our squad car so we could talk to them. As we walked out the door the two suddenly sprinted away, running in separate directions. I chased one of them on foot and had run approximately a block full-out (which is harder than it sounds--try it sometime) when I tired and tripped, falling to the pavement and ripping my pant leg. When I righted myself the suspect was long gone and I was left empty-handed, embarrassed, and peeved with myself for not being in better shape. When I returned to the store I found out the other suspect had outrun my partner and also escaped. We searched the car in which the two had arrived and found it to be stolen and to contain two Halloween masks and two sawed-off shotguns. The suspects hadn't been petty thieves, they'd been armed robbers (or planned to be)! Now I was really angry with myself and vowed to never take a call for granted and to never lose a foot chase again (or at least to be competitive). I started running.

By 1989 I was in better shape and had won more foot chases than I had lost. I was, indeed, competitive. I had been running 5-mile and 10-kilometer runs and ran several times a week. Then one day my knee gave out on me. I could walk fine but when I tried to run the jolting on the knee made it give out. I could run short distances but could no longer run far enough to keep in shape. I had to find some other way to stay healthy and active. Racquetball helped but I needed something I could do without someone else so I could do it every day and not have to arrange a time and court.

I had an old Schwinn 10-speed bicycle in the garage from years before and thought I'd give it a try. The tires were flat so I wheeled it down to the local gas station and proceeded to blow the inner tube by putting too much air in the first tire I tried to fill (the tubes fill up fast using a power air pump). So I sheepishly wheeled the bike to the local bike shop and got the tire fixed. You might say I was a bit discouraged; but riding the bike home made me feel better and I decided to give bike riding (I didn't call it cycling back then) a chance. I thought five miles would be a pretty good test so I drove the car two-and-a-half miles from home and back to get a five-mile route set in my head. I then rode the five miles, assuming that I would be pretty exhausted when I returned, and was surprised to find that five miles isn't that far on a bike. I started riding seven to ten miles at a time several times a week and on one particularly pleasant ride (good weather, country scenery, birds chirping, wind in the trees) thought, "I can't believe more people don't do this!" I was hooked.

I now average 2500 miles a year on the bike, which isn't considered very many in cycling circles (but, c'mon, get a life!) and I consider myself a serious-casual rider. I still play racquetball, tennis, and ski but if I were forced to give up one form of exercise, it wouldn't be cycling. It is a great low-impact, pleasant exercise and a great way to see the countryside or cityscape close up and still cover a lot of ground. I ride shorter rides (15-20 miles) for exercise several days a week and longer rides (50-90 miles) occasionally. Each year I take two week-long rides (300-400 miles)--one an organized ride where the sponsors of the ride carry my gear (clothing and tent) and one with two or three friends in which we carry our gear in bags, called panniers, attached to our bikes. I have upgraded to a Trek 1000 road bike (which is now twenty years old) and a Trek 7500 hybrid bike (for the week-long carry-everything-with-me rides or light off-road riding). I have no plans to replace either of them soon as they are both "running like new."

Please keep in mind while reading this book that I <u>in no way whatsoever</u> claim to be an expert on cycling. I am trying to accomplish two things: Encourage people to give cycling a chance and answer some of the questions that arise before they start or are still in the early stages of riding. The topics I will cover come from questions I have been asked many times by friends or people who have just found out that I am a cyclist. If you bought this book thinking otherwise, please pass it on to a friend and do not, under any circumstances, take it back to where you bought it for a full refund. Much of what I write here is my opinion and things that I have found to be true through experience. If someone disagrees with or thinks they can "disprove" something I've written, they can write their own book.

To get across the point of how enjoyable cycling can be (it can be unpleasant at times, too, but that's a subject for a different book) I include, at the end of each chapter, a short (or not) story about an experience I would not have had, a sight I would not have seen, or a person I would not have met if I had not taken up cycling. These stories are marked **ANECDOTE** because that just sounds better than "story."

And here is a caveat for you: Sometimes cycling can be unpleasant--but if you are going to see the great view from the top of the hill you will first have to put in some serious pedal-time. Some days it will be too hot, too windy, too hilly or, after you have ridden a while and are still an hour from home, it will start to rain. Nothing's perfect. I like to say that cycling is a good life-lesson--sometimes you have to work to get to the good stuff and sometimes the good stuff is even better because you had to work to get there.

Chapter 1
Getting Started

Let me start out by saying this: This is a book for people who think they may want to take up bicycling again as an adult for exercise and recreation. If you are a put-your-head-down-and-ride-like-the-wind-while-only-seeing-the-pavement-and-the-tire-in-front-of-you cyclist quit reading this book now and pick up a cycling magazine (I hear there is a good article on "Expectorating in a Pace Line" in one of them).

So--you found the old bicycle gathering dust (and other stuff) in the back of the garage, remembered how you used to enjoy riding around the neighborhood on warm spring days, and are now contemplating renewing the experience. You have a bit more time on your hands, have realized, after years of running the race, that sometimes slower and less complicated are better, and are looking for a pleasant, low-impact way of getting some exercise. Or maybe you've seen the people on bikes riding the trails and roadways around you and just think it looks like fun.

Whatever the reason, cycling has come into your consciousness and you are wondering how to start. Good for you--good start. Now what? Do you need one of those new, feather-light, expensive, 21-gear, Lance Armstrong-type bicycles you see being ridden by brightly-dressed, steel-legged, Lance Armstrong-type cyclists on the road each day? Or should you opt for one of the expensive, knobby-tired, heavy-duty, dirt-taming, mountain bikes you see on the tops of 4-wheel-drive SUV's on the freeways whose owners are obviously on their way to a wilderness adventure? Maybe you should just get the department store bike because it's cheap and brightly-colored and looks about the same as the others anyway. I've got three words for you---no, no, no!

Let me give some credentials here. While I in no way claim to be a cycling "expert," I have done quite a bit of cycling, and feel that some of my experience could be beneficial to someone looking to take up cycling. As I write this I am in my late-50's, in reasonably good shape (notice I did not say, "...for my age"), and have been cycling (as an adult) for twenty years.

TRAM (The Ride Across Minnesota), Multiple Sclerosis Society's annual ride, was my first week-long ride and was (and still is) an excellent ride for a novice as the organizers take such good care of the riders.

That year I started keeping track of my mileage and ended up riding 800 miles. I now average 2500 miles a season (which, in cycling circles, gets me just into the serious-casual class), have done numerous cross-state rides, and do one organized week-long bike ride (one sponsored and supported by an organization) with hundreds of other cyclists and one week-long, carry-all-your-gear-with-you-on-the-bike ride with a couple of friends each year. But enough about me.

So what do you do when you think you might want to get into this cycling thing? The first thing to do is curb your enthusiasm; don't buy that new bike yet. Find out if you really want to do this or if it will be a good fit for you. Fill the tires of the old bike (if you do this at a gas station be careful; it is easy to over-inflate them as the small tubes fill up fast--a floor hand-pump is a better option) and spend a couple of hours (not all at once) riding around the neighborhood to see if your memories of enjoyment are correct. Maybe even put the bike in the van and take it to a bike trail to get the feel of riding through the countryside without the worry of traffic. Don't have an old bike? Try renting one on vacation or going to a trail with a rental shop close and rent a good-quality bike. But keep in mind that a fat tire beach bicycle is not what you would ride around the neighborhood so would not be a good way to find out if you like cycling.

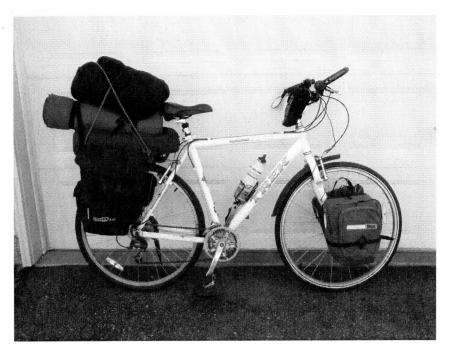

Author's bicycle loaded for a week long self-supported ride.

Start out with short distances. Try a couple of miles first and see how you feel (and see how you feel the next day). If, after a short trial period, you decide you do want to pursue this particular activity, you can decide how you want to approach it. If the old bike is a quality bike (even though it's old) you probably don't have to buy a new one--a tune-up will do. If the old bike just isn't going to cut it, however, start looking for a new one.

But the most important thing is to actually do it; quit talking about it, thinking about it, contemplating it, or talking about the possibility of thinking about maybe contemplating it and go out and do it! It's not that difficult; just do it.

Anecdote

After riding The Ride Across Minnesota five times my friend, Eric, and I decided we could do our own week-long ride carrying our clothing in panniers (bags) attached to our bikes. Wanting to see something other than the Midwest, we planned a ride in Vermont and Upstate New York, starting and ending in Burlington, VT, circling Lake Champlain, with a side trip to Lake Placid, NY.

We flew into Albany, NY and drove to Burlington with a stop-over in Rochester, VT to rent bikes from Green Mt. Bicycles owned by Doon Hinderyckx, "The Biking Viking." This was one of our best trips ever; we saw Fort Ticonderoga, the Olympic Training site in Lake Placid, rode the Olympic bobsled ride (on rollers, of course) at Mount Hoevenberg, took the boat trip through the Ausable Chasm, swam in very refreshing, if very cold, Lake Champlain, and, of course, rode through beautiful countryside.

But my favorite memory of the trip occurred after a long (70 miles), hot day riding through the mountains from Lake Placid to Elizabethtown, NY. At the end of the day we had to climb a long, steep mountain pass, then coast into Elizabethtown, a town of about 800 people. We got a room at the Park Motor Inn and asked the proprietor if there were a municipal swimming pool in town. To our vast disappointment, as the thought of a cool swim had been on our minds as we climbed the pass, he told us there was none. After a moment's thought, though, he told us we could try the swimming hole the town's youth use and gave us directions which entailed going back up the road a mile (just past an abandoned car), looking for a large culvert pipe next to a small gravel parking area, and looking over the far edge of the parking area. We followed the directions and were delighted to see, upon looking over the edge, a small swimming hole about twenty feet below. It was about twelve feet deep with water so clear we could see the bottom. We enjoyed the cool water for a half-hour or so and were sitting on the bank enjoying the shade when we heard, but could not see, a car pull into the parking area above. Two car doors slammed and seconds later two figures launched themselves from the parking area and plunged into the pool. The town's youth had begun to arrive. This happened several more times as we sat there. We quickly figured that we could tell how many figures would be plunging by how many car doors we heard slam. We at first worried that someone in the pool would get hit by one of the plunging teens but noticed that when the car doors slammed anyone in the pool would swim away from the middle where the plungers invariably would splash down. We assumed that slamming the car door loudly and hitting the middle of the pool was an unwritten rule.

Later that evening we found a wonderful little restaurant, The Deer's Head Inn, for a gourmet dinner and, the next morning, played a quick nine holes at the Cobble Hill Golf Course before riding off for Vermont. All in all, it was a great stop.

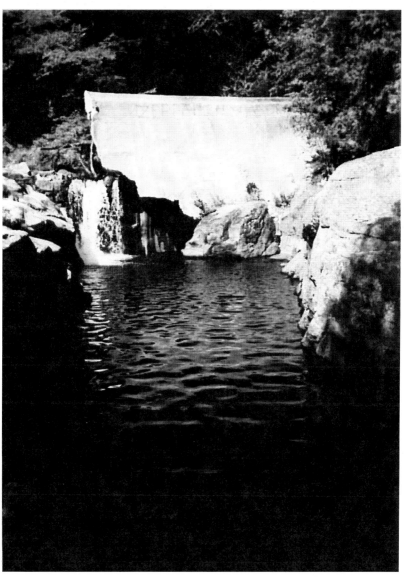

The swimming hole in Upstate New York

Chapter 2
Buying the Bike

Many people think they have to buy an expensive bicycle right away and end up with an expensive garage-wall ornament. I tell people a moderately-priced shiny new bike will look just as good hanging on the garage wall as an expensive shiny new bike and suggest they buy the moderately-priced one. A moderately-priced bicycle will suffice most people looking to get back into cycling for at least several years and probably quite a bit longer. You can get a quality cycle for less than you might think--somewhere in the $400 range. And the price is easier to swallow if you realize the bike won't wear out for years; I've had my Trek 1000 for twenty years now (I was told by a bike store owner that it almost qualifies as an antique) and it still works just fine. And a friend of mine still rides the same bike he had as a teenager (he's my age, by the way). Spend more if you wish but don't think that you have to.

So what kind of bicycle should you buy? There are three main kinds of bicycles--road bikes, mountain bikes, and hybrids or cross-bikes.

Mountain Bikes

Mountain bikes have handlebars that go straight across (rather than curl under like a road bike) and wide, knobby tires that are good for extreme off-road riding but create too much friction for riding pavement or even light off-road riding such as crushed limestone or packed dirt bike trails. They also may have suspension systems that make riding streets more difficult. You will probably pay a good deal of money for features that won't help, and may even harm, your riding experience. I always advise people away from a mountain bike (because of the friction factor) unless they are planning on actually doing extreme off-road riding. Over the years I have had many people tell me they regretted getting a mountain bike because of the difficulty of pedaling and the "singing" noise the tires make on the pavement.

Road Bikes

If you decide on a road bike you have to choose between the faster, racing-style bike or the touring-style bike. If you don't plan on riding on anything but pavement the racing-style bike with the narrow, high-pressure tires is a good choice as the tires create less friction and the bike rolls easier. It may seem as if one would get better exercise by pedaling harder but that is not the case. The good exercise comes from pedaling faster (more revolutions), not pedaling harder. Pedaling harder, that is, more forcefully, is just harder on the knees. If you are planning on riding eighty to a hundred miles at a time as fast as you can this is the bike for you. Keep in mind, though, that the narrow tires don't handle adverse conditions (loose gravel or sand, wet leaves, etc.) well and the rider must take care when leaving pavement for another surface. Most people just getting back into cycling aren't doing it for the speed or the challenge, though; they're doing it for the enjoyment and exercise. A touring bike isn't as fast or as light as the racing bike but it gives a more steady ride so if you think you will ride on dirt bike trails or gravel roads from time-to-time the touring bike with the slightly wider tires would be a better choice.

Both racing and the touring bikes have the "curled under" style handlebar which make the rider lean forward a bit more, putting a bit more weight on the palms of the hands and causing the rider to flex the neck muscles to keep the head up.

Hybrids

Hybrids are a cross between a mountain bike and a road bike with tires wider than a road bike but narrower than a mountain bike. They also have handlebars like a mountain bike so the rider sits more upright than on a road bike.

I personally think the hybrid is more comfortable as you don't have to bend over the handlebars so far and, as you are more upright, don't have to strain your neck keeping your head up. It is also easier to look around at the scenery (which is, after all, one of the reasons you're out there), and the wider tires handle dirt trails or shoulders better while not slowing you down too much.

Recumbents

These are those "barca-lounger bikes" which allow the rider to sit in what looks like a lounge chair. They are very comfortable as the seat is much larger than a regular bike's seat and the rider's hands and arms don't take the punishment that comes with leaning on the handlebars. However, they are also expensive, take some getting used to, and are harder to transport, so I don't advise someone just starting out to get one.

Fit

Once you have decided what style and price range is right for you the staff at the bicycle store will fit you with the right size bicycle. It is important that the bike fit your body--another reason to buy the bike at a bike store and not just buy one "off the rack." The distance between the seat and the handlebars is very important for comfort, as is the height of the bike. Again, bike store staff will be able to help you get the right fit. If the person selling the bike doesn't talk about fit get another sales person or go to a different store.

If you are going to use the old bike make sure it fits you. You should be able to stand astride the top tube with both feet flat on the ground. When sitting on the bike with a foot on the pedal you should be able to extend your leg almost to its fullest, but with a slight bend at the knee. There's more to a good fit than this, of course (see Ch. 8), but this is a good start. If you buy a new bike or take the old one for a tune-up, have the bike shop employee help you get the proper fit.

EQUIPMENT

Whether you're going to buy a new bike or make do with the old one, buy a helmet and wear it. If you're buying a new bike you might as well get a water bottle carrier and bottle right away. You'll want to take water with you as you ride and the carrier and bottle are cheap. I'll go further into equipment in a later chapter (aptly named "Equipment").

DECIDING

Don't make the decision on which bike to buy too difficult. Years ago a co-worker came to me looking for advice on buying bikes. He said he and his girlfriend were going to get bikes and said, somewhat derisively, "When I asked her what kind of bikes we should buy she said she wants red ones."

He then pulled out a chart on which he had obviously spent quite a bit of time. He had listed three different brands of bicycles, all of them quality bikes, and had meticulously itemized the components (brakes, shifters, drive train) of each and was comparing the bikes in an attempt to get the best buy. He showed me his chart, explained his system of comparisons, and asked me which bikes I thought they should buy. Without hesitation I answered, "The red ones."

He had made the purchase way too complicated. All three bikes were quality bikes and any of them would have quality components. I told him they should ride the bikes, see which of them felt best to them, and buy that one.

Anecdote

In 1998 three friends and I rode a weeklong ride from St. Paul, MN to Dubuque, IA along The Great River Road (which follows the Mississippi River) and planned to stop at Iowa's Effigy Mounds National Monument, past which I had planned our route. It was late in the day and raining as we arrived so we decided to ride the three miles into the nearest town, Marquette, IA, get rooms for the night, and return the next day.

We stayed the night at The Frontier Motel and in the morning, as it was still misting, decided to catch a taxi to the monument so we wouldn't get wet just getting to the site. I went to the front desk, explained our idea to one of the owners of the motel, and asked if there were any local taxis. The owner, Sally Kann, said, "Just take our car, we won't need it for a while." and handed me the keys to her and her husband's new car. She was willing to let four strangers use her new car so they wouldn't have to pay for a cab. You have to love small-town America. We filled the car's tank (gas was cheaper then) in appreciation and Sally admonished us saying, "You didn't have to do that."

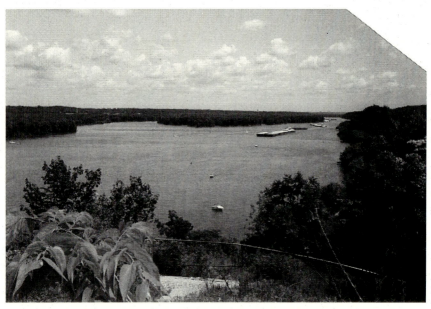

On The Great River Road outside Dubuque, Iowa.

Chapter 3
Starting to Ride

Now that you have either fixed up the old bike or bought a new one, you are ready to hit the trail and start reaping the benefits of cycling. Great, you won't regret it. There are some things you should know as you start your new regimen of fitness and fun.

When friends or new acquaintances find out that I ride bicycle semi-seriously they often comment that they have considered cycling for exercise and enjoyment but just aren't sure how to go about doing it. They wonder how long the rides should be, what equipment is necessary, where they should go to ride (trails or roads), and other questions that aren't terribly important in and of themselves, but, when combined, tend to discourage getting started.

One of the good things about cycling is you can do it right from your home. While loading the bike on the car or in the van and taking it to a park or bike trail is certainly a nice option, it is by no means necessary. City streets and county roads make for excellent riding and can be reached easily on the bike (they're at the end of your driveway). While big city streets and heavily-traveled roads are a bit tricky and should be avoided whenever possible, they shouldn't keep you from getting to less busy roads. I lived in a high-rise apartment building in downtown St. Paul, Minn. (which has a great trail system) for a year and enjoyed numerous bike trails that could be reached with only a few minutes of riding in traffic. Unless you are planning a longer ride (more than an hour) the time and energy used to pack up the bike and drive to a trail can often be better used by just biking around the neighborhood. In many cases the bike trail to which you are going can be reached by bike if you factor the time to-and-from into your biking time. And riding around the neighborhood has another benefit--you discover things (houses, parks, gardens, neighbors) that you never get a chance to, or have reason to, pass in your car.

Another good thing about cycling is that you don't have to be on track for an Olympic medal to get exercise. Don't be discouraged when other cyclists (some of whom look as if they are, indeed, on track for a medal) pass you. It isn't a race, there is no trophy; you are out there for you, no one else. As long as you are getting exercise and enjoying it you <u>are</u> winning.

Traffic Laws

Obey all traffic laws. According to the Minnesota Dept. of Transportation bicycles have all the rights and responsibilities of a motor vehicle, including the right to operate in a traffic lane and ride in the roadway. Cyclists must stop at stop signs and stop lights, signal turns, ride with the flow of traffic, never against it, and ride as far to the right of the roadway as practicable. Cyclists are allowed to ride two abreast in a driving lane but should move to single-file to allow faster traffic to pass. Motorists must at all times maintain a three-foot clearance when passing a bicycle and, when a motor vehicle is overtaking a bicycle, the bicycle has the right-of-way. Check the traffic laws in your own state but I believe that most states have similar laws. Ride courteously; treat motorists as you want to be treated when you are driving. Not long ago I was driving a main street in my area and came upon two cyclists riding side-by-side, one on the shoulder and one in the driving lane. The street was one with a driving lane in each direction and a center, "Left Turn Only" lane. The car in front of me had to go into the "Left Turn Only" lane to pass them (in Minnesota it's illegal to pass in the "Left Turn Only" lane) and as I approached I tapped on my horn once to let the cyclist in the driving lane know I was approaching hoping he would move to single file. The cyclist did not move, however, even though it would have been easy to do, and I had to pass him illegally (or hold up other traffic). Keep in mind that while cyclists do have the right to be in the roadway, the roads were built for faster, larger vehicles. Also be aware that some motorists just don't like cyclists in the roadway whatever the law says and just plain refuse to share the road. Watch out for them.

HELMET

This bears repeating--buy one, wear it! I know it isn't cool looking but it is an item you should wear at all times while riding. That being said, let me say this--when you stop at the local coffee shop or drive-in for a well-deserved break, TAKE THE HELMET OFF! When you're riding you have an excuse, but when you're sitting on a stool in an establishment you look positively dorky wearing your helmet. I know it's hard to find a place to set it but you figured out where to put your cell phone, blackberry, and laptop--find a place for the helmet. As far as I know no one has ever suffered a head injury while sipping a double-mocha latte with cinnamon sprinkles and just a touch of vanilla (although I suppose that could make one a bit woozy).

WHERE TO RIDE

For the most part there are two choices of where to ride--a roadway or a bike trail. A mountain bike trail usually will not work for anything other than a mountain bike. Try not to use sidewalks unless you absolutely have to.

ROADWAYS

When riding on a roadway ride on the right side of the road, with (in the same direction as) traffic, just as if you were on a small motor scooter. This lessens "closing time" allowing motor vehicle drivers more time to see and react to your presence and would lessen damage (to you) if, heaven forbid, a vehicle were to hit you. Pedestrians should walk facing traffic but cyclists should ride with traffic. In Minnesota cyclists have the right to ride on the roadway, except freeways (some states do allow freeway riding), but common sense and courtesy should prevail here. According to the Minnesota Department of Transportation cyclists may ride two abreast but should ride "...as far to the right as practicable." If you happen on a one-way street you can use lanes the same as if you were in a motor vehicle. Of course, if you can stay on the shoulder out of the way of motor vehicles you should do so but you do have the right to be in a driving lane. That does not, however, mean that it is always safe or smart to do so--but you will have to make that determination. I always cringe when I see a person pulling a toddler-trailer containing a child or two behind their bike on a busy, high-speed highway.

BIKE TRAILS

When riding a bike trail stay to the right of the trail. If you are with a friend and riding side-by-side move to single file around corners or when going up a hill. Remember that there will be other riders on the trail. If two cyclists riding side-by-side over a hill meet two other cyclists riding side-by-side over the same hill in the opposite direction, the enjoyment of at least two of the cyclists could be greatly curtailed.

Most states or municipalities outlaw riding on sidewalks because of the possibility of bicycle/pedestrian collisions. Beyond that, cyclists should be discouraged from riding on the sidewalk as motorists are not expecting a bicyclist, moving much faster than a pedestrian, to cross the street in a crosswalk. But if for some reason you have to use a sidewalk for a short time (very heavy road traffic, for instance) slow down and do it carefully. If there are pedestrians on the sidewalk get off the bike and walk it until you can get back onto the trail or roadway. If you are riding on a trail or sidewalk on the side of the street that faces oncoming traffic, remember that as drivers approach on a cross-street they are not accustomed to looking to their right for traffic when turning right. And some drivers driving parallel to the cyclist may not see him or her when turning onto a cross-street, thus turning in front of the cyclist. It is up to you, for your safety, to make sure that a driver in that situation sees you coming. For the most part, though, avoid riding on sidewalks at all.

I've noticed that we cyclists have the tendency, especially after a long day of riding, to think that we are the only ones out there. Riding can be somewhat mesmerizing; we can forget there are many other vehicles for which we need to be alert, both for our own good and for theirs. Try not to fall into this trap, be vigilant for traffic and conditions that could cause problems.

Remember the trails are multi-use. Cyclists share them with walkers, in-line skaters (who can be hard to pass as they are often wearing earphones and don't hear you announce yourself), and other non-cyclists. If you are going to stop for a moment, don't do so in the middle of the trail--you are not the only one out there. It is easy, especially after some time of riding through the countryside, to forget that the trail crosses roadways, keep an eye out for crossings so you don't ride right into traffic.

BRAKING

With hand brakes you want to use the rear brake (right brake lever) more than the front brake. Using the front brake too heavily can cause you to pitch forward and lose your balance. Get used to using both at the same time, using the front brake more lightly than the rear brake. If you have to brake hard, use the rear brake and don't lean forward. If you have to perform an "emergency brake," push yourself as far back as you can on the bike while you brake. Don't brake while standing as it is easy to lose your balance or pitch forward over the handlebars.

CURVES

When you take a curve at a bit faster speed keep the pedal on the side to which you are leaning in the "up" position. If the pedal is in the "down" position it can make contact with the pavement giving you a nasty jolt and throwing you off balance. Control your speed on a downhill curve; it is easy to misjudge the curve and ride out of your lane or off the trail.

Announce Yourself

When overtaking a pedestrian or another cyclist (yes, some people will be even slower than you are) "announce" your approach with a bell, pleasant greeting ("Good morning." works well, depending on the time of day), or by saying, "On your left." well before you pass. To zip past someone who may very well take a side-step into your path not knowing you are approaching is discourteous and can be dangerous for both of you. And remember that many people will jump and side-step one way or the other when you first announce your presence, so do it well before you are actually going to pass. I've been walking on paths (all-purpose paths) and had cyclists go past so quietly, closely, and quickly that if I had stepped or even leaned to the side at the wrong time we both would have been injured. And it usually isn't the Olympic hopefuls doing that, it's the casual rider (or so their blue jean and flannel riding attire would make it seem).

Motorists

This one is a no-brainer but I see it happen from time-to-time (and have done it myself in the heat of the moment). Don't get into arguments with drivers. The dual-carb, twin-cam, 4 X 4 Ram Charger with a hemi is a lot bigger and faster than we are and, in this case, guys, size really does matter.

Earphones

Don't wear earphones, you need to hear some things (traffic, other cyclists, etc.) while other things (birds, wind in the trees, etc.) are nice to hear. Do we really need to be electronically entertained all the time? I do some of my best thinking while riding (sometimes I rides and thinks and sometimes I just rides).

Ride in a Straight Line

Riding in a straight line let's others know what you are doing. If you weave back and forth as you ride motorists will have trouble knowing where you are going or what your intentions are. And anyone riding next to you will have to be constantly ready to veer out of your way and if they do have to veer around you they may have to ride into someone else's path. Ride in a straight line.

Signal Your Turns

Just as when you're driving a car, signaling your turns is important. Letting motorists and other cyclists know your intentions is courteous to them and safer for you. Get into the habit of signaling; do it even when there is no other traffic. If you get into the habit you will eventually do it automatically, and, conversely, if you don't get into the habit, you'll forget to do it when there is traffic around. You already know the signals--point to the left with your left arm for a left turn and hold your left arm out with the arm bent up at the elbow for a right turn. It is also acceptable to point to the right with your right arm for a right turn. Hold the left hand down with the palm facing back to indicate you are going to slow down or stop. However you do it, let others know what you intend to do.

Railroad Tracks

Cross railroad tracks at a right angle. If your tire drops into the groove alongside the rail your bike <u>will</u> stop--and you won't. If the tracks don't cross the road at a right angle, adjust your approach so you cross the tracks at a right angle.

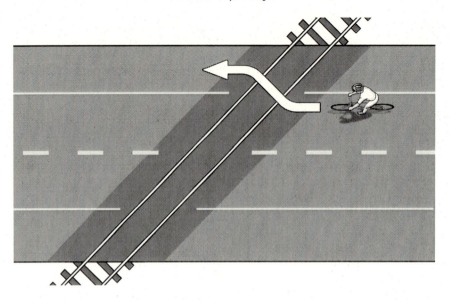

RIDING IN THE DARK

Don't. There's no reason to ride at night when you are just starting out. You can't see debris in the roadway and at motor vehicle speeds it is difficult for drivers to realize what you are and react accordingly even if you do have all the proper lighting on the bike. I'm surprised and dismayed at how often I see a person on a bicycle alongside a busy highway at night with no lights or reflectors on the bike and wearing dark clothing. Those people must have a death wish! If you must ride at night, wait to do so until you are quite comfortable riding in traffic and varying conditions. See Chapter 9 on More Serious Riding.

CLOTHING

Always wear bright-colored clothing, especially in low-light conditions (dusk, rain, clouds, dark). Don't get hung up on looking like a "cyclist." You'll find as you ride more that spandex is nice because it doesn't chafe, but when you first start out you probably won't be going that far or that fast so clothing won't make that much difference. Blue jeans should be avoided, however, as the chafing factor is pretty high. Shorts of some kind and a t-shirt will do fine. On colder days sweat pants will work as long as you put something around the right pant leg to keep it from getting caught in the chain. Tennis shoes also work fine but do something to keep the laces out of the chain.

INTERSECTIONS

There are a couple of ways to handle intersections depending on the type of intersection, traffic control devices (stop signs, red lights, right turn lanes), and traffic congestion. Remember that you are a vehicle and as such have all the responsibility of a motor vehicle. At uncontrolled intersections you have to yield to the vehicle to your right, just as if you were driving a car. Keep in mind that a bicycle is not as easy to see as a motor vehicle so cars that should yield to you may not do so (either because the drivers don't see you or because the drivers think you have no right-of-way).

At controlled intersections, especially busy ones, the easiest way to cross is to just go to the crosswalk, wait for the light to change or for your turn at the stop sign, and cross in the crosswalk. Be sure to watch for vehicles turning right at the intersection. This is the easiest, safest way to cross and if you have children riding with you I recommend it.

An adult rider, however, will understandably become impatient with this method and will want a quicker way to cross that doesn't include dismounting. If you are just going straight or turning right it is fairly easy to just stay to one side of the lane, stop for the stop sign or signal (if necessary), and continue through the intersection. This can become complicated, however, when there is a right turn lane (and you are not turning right), traffic is heavy, or you have to make a left turn. These situations will be covered in Chapter 9, "More Serious Riding."

CROSSWALKS

While you are on the bicycle you are a vehicle, not a pedestrian. If we want all the rights of a vehicle we can't expect to be treated like pedestrians just because we ride into a crosswalk. If you want to be a pedestrian, get off the bike and walk into the crosswalk, otherwise, act as if you are in a car and yield to traffic going past until such a time that you can cross safely. Recently, while I was driving my car, I watched an older rider riding with traffic, coming at me on the opposite side of the street. As she approached a crosswalk in the middle of the street that led from a park to a beach she suddenly turned left (with no signal) from the street into the crosswalk and rode directly in front of me. I had to slam on my brakes to avoid hitting her. She gave me a dirty look and I'm certain she thought she was right because she was in a crosswalk, but she had actually turned left in front of me without signaling and failed to yield. If I had not seen her on the other side of the road as we approached each other I am certain I would have hit her. A crosswalk does not give a cyclist the right to ride into a traffic lane any more than it gives a pedestrian the right to dash into a line of traffic.

RIGHT-TURN LANES

Right-turn lanes can be a bit tricky. If the rider who wants to go straight ahead stays to the far right of the lane, motorists will think he is going to turn right. If the rider stays in the middle of the lane vehicles approaching from the rear will have to wait or go around and then get back into the lane. I find the best way to handle the right-turn lane is to stay in the far left of the lane so it is more obvious that I am going straight ahead. A car turning right can go to the right of me and a car in the traffic lane still has room to pass.

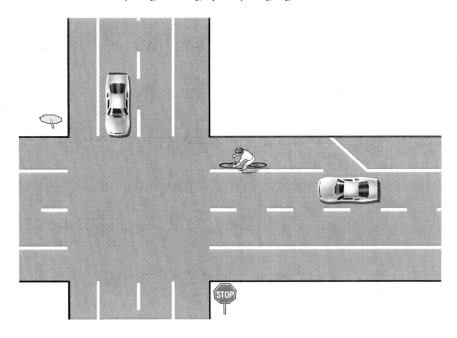

Fortunately, most right-turn lanes are short so won't cause a problem for very long, if at all. Some right-turn lanes are wider than others and if the one you are in at the time is narrow I would suggest staying in the middle and let a car behind you wait the couple of seconds it will take you to get past the lane.

Dogs

Eventually, you will get chased by a dog. While most dogs, in my experience, don't mean you any harm, they can cause it by getting in front of you and tipping you over. This has never happened to me, by the way, but it is possible. Most of the time the dog just wants to chase you. There are various options for handling dogs and you can decide which one is right for the particular incident. Dogs sense fear so try to stay calm. You can stop and get off the bike quickly, using the bike for a shield, and walk away. The dog may lose interest in you once the thrill of the chase is over (sound familiar, ladies?). If the dog attacks, use the bike as a shield and yell scary things like, "Bad dog!" and, "No!" and, "Go home!" in a firm (scary) voice. Carry a whistle with you and blow it at the dog as you are riding or squirt water from your water bottle at him. Many times the dog will stop as the noise or the water startles him. I don't recommend pepper spray as it has a nasty habit of blowing back into the user's face and is hard to keep on the bike without contaminating whatever is near it.

ANECDOTE

In 1999, the year after the St. Paul to Dubuque ride, my friends and I rode from Dubuque to St. Louis along the Mississippi River (again on the Great River Road). On our last day of riding we found ourselves on the wrong side of the Mississippi River and realized the only way to get into St. Louis was over a freeway bridge which we assumed would be illegal and dangerous. We stopped at a convenience store in Hartford, Ill. to get information about a crossing but as we rode up saw a sign that read "Open Next Month." As we were about to leave a motorist pulled into the lot and gave us directions to an open store that consisted of, "Go down this street three blocks and turn left--it's just a block from there." We thanked the motorist and rode off. All four of us rode three blocks and turned <u>right</u> and did not realize our mistake for about two blocks by which time we were in front of the Hartford Ribs Smokehouse and Bakery. As it was lunchtime anyway we decided to have a sandwich and hopefully get some help with our dilemma. We explained the situation to one of the owners, Chris Shewmaker (who was making our sandwiches), and she said, "The old Chain-of-Rocks highway bridge is open for bikes but only on weekends. But if you wait a couple of minutes Deanna, who works for the city, will be in for lunch and she may know more." We waited, hoping Deanna hadn't taken the day off, and several minutes later Chris said, "There she is across the street. She'll go into the store to get her bottle of milk and then come over here for her sandwich." Sure enough, a minute later a lady emerged from the store carrying a small bottle of milk, crossed the street, and entered the shop. After hearing our story, Deanna Barnes, who was the administrative assistant and projects manager for the city of Hartford, told us the bridge was open to bikes and pedestrians on weekends but was locked on weekdays (this was a weekday, of course). She called "Gene," who held a similar position in a nearby city and who had a key for the gate to the bridge. Gene (whose last name I don't know but whose photo is in one of my albums) met us at the bridge, opened the gate, followed *us across the bridge, opened the gate on the other side, then followed us for a mile-and-a-half in his van (with flashers on) down a busy road which led to a bike trail. We thanked him profusely and went on our way. Ten miles later the bike trail ended at the foot of St. Louis' Gateway Arch and our ride was complete. Once again we had been lucky--if we had not stopped at the closed store, messed up the directions, and stopped at the sandwich shop at Deanna's lunchtime we would have never found out about, much less gotten to use, the Chain-of-Rocks Bridge. Luck and the kindness of strangers had once again saved the day.*

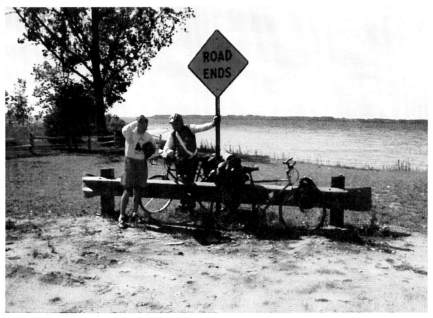

The best laid routes of mice and men...

Chapter 4
Shifting

I felt shifting was important enough to warrant its own chapter.

Learn to Shift

One of the things I tell people is to learn to shift. While there are older-style one speed bikes and bikes with automatic shifting, most bikes come with numerous (eighteen to twenty-one) gears and need to be shifted by the rider. Don't be intimidated by the number of gears; you only need three or four of them most of the time and the shifters are right on the handlebars, or even the handgrips, making it easy to shift. Shifting allows the rider to maintain pedal revolution pace when conditions change and to increase speed without a corresponding increase in effort. You don't want to ride up a steep hill in the same gear you ride downhill or on level ground. Conditions change constantly and if you don't shift you are going to be pedaling too fast (while moving slowly) or pedaling too slowly (and with difficulty). I have often seen a novice rider struggling mightily up a hill that could have been ridden fairly easily (or at least easier) if the rider had just shifted down a gear or two.

Older bikes work on a "friction" system which makes the rider listen while shifting and decide when the chain is in the proper spot. If the chain is not quite in the gear, the chain will make an annoying "rattling" sound and the rider will have to adjust the shifter until the sound abates. Newer bikes have an "index" system in which the chain moves to the gear immediately when the shifter is moved to the gear number. This provides a satisfying "click" sound each time the rider shifts to another gear and eliminates the "rattling."

Front Sprockets

There are three sprockets (gears) on the front of the chain, right at the pedals--a small one (the "granny-gear"), a mid-sized one, and a large one. The small sprocket makes it very easy to pedal (thus the name) and is usually only used for going up hills. On flat or downhill terrain it will be too easy to pedal this gear, making your legs spin too fast and the tires spin too slowly. The large sprocket makes it harder to pedal (and increases speed) and is used when the rider has built up speed in the middle sprocket and wants to increase speed even more. This gear is useful when the rider is going downhill and wants to keep pedaling--if the rider stays in the middle sprocket his or her legs will spin too fast and will not be able to keep up with the pedals' revolutions. This gear also works well on flat terrain if the rider gradually works up speed, then shifts. The middle sprocket is, obviously, mid-range and I do most of my riding in this gear. The front sprockets are controlled by the left-hand shifter.

As the front sprockets are bigger, you have to move the left shifter farther to move the gears than you do using the right shifter. Shifting moves the angle of the chain slightly and sometimes shifting a rear gear will cause the chain to rub against the front derailleur (mechanism that guides the chain) causing a "rattling" sound as you pedal. Moving the left shifter a "click" or two will move the front derailleur slightly, alleviating the noise without changing the gears.

Rear Sprockets

In the rear of the bike, attached to the rear wheel, are six or seven smaller sprockets of various sizes controlled by the right-hand shifter. These work the opposite of the front sprockets--the smaller the gear (sprocket), the harder it is to pedal in that gear.

I usually leave the chain in the middle front sprocket and shift the rear sprockets to fit riding conditions. When starting out, put the chain in the middle front and rear sprockets and shift the rear sprockets until it is comfortable to pedal, so it isn't so easy that your legs are spinning uncomfortably fast or so hard that it is a strain to pedal. Now practice shifting the front and rear gears up and down as you ride around the neighborhood until it becomes comfortable. The chain needs to be in motion to move up or down the sprockets so pedal as you shift. Try the different combinations of gears; shift to the "granny-gear" in front and up and down the rear sprockets, then do the same with the middle and large front sprockets noticing the variations. Before shifting "up" a gear in front shift "down" to a lower gear in back so the change won't be so drastic. Remember that in front the bigger the sprocket the higher the gear but in back the <u>smaller</u> the sprocket the higher the gear. This means to shift "down" in the rear sprockets you'll be moving the chain "up" the sprockets. Try not to ponder this too much--you shouldn't be looking back at the rear sprockets anyway as you might miss the fact that a car just stopped in front of you. As you practice you'll find your comfort zone and learn when it is comfortable for you to shift from one gear to the next (you may not have to shift all the way down in the rear gears to shift up comfortably in front).

Again, you probably won't need all the gears very often, but it will be good to know that you can get into the gears if necessary.

WHEN TO SHIFT

This isn't rocket science or brain surgery or, as a friend of mine likes to say, rocket surgery. Whatever, don't make it harder than it is. When it gets too easy to pedal, when your legs are spinning too fast and you're having trouble keeping up with the pedals' revolutions, shift up. When the pedaling is hard, shift down. Let's go over that again. Pedaling too easy--shift up, pedaling too hard--shift down. If you've shifted as low as you can and the pedaling is still too hard, get off the bike and walk it to the top of the mountain--walking is good for you, too. Except on hills, the pedaling should always be fairly easy, the exercise comes from the revolutions, not the difficulty of pushing the pedals down. Riding in too high a gear, forcing the rider to push down hard on the pedals, is hard on the knees.

If you shift into higher gears as you pick up speed, remember to shift back down when you are slowing or coming to a stop so you don't have to start up again in a high gear.

Shifting on Hills

Knowing how to shift can really help, and, in fact, is often absolutely necessary while climbing hills. A long, gradual hill, a short, steep hill, or worse, a long, steep hill poses a problem--pedaling is going to be harder, maybe a lot harder. If you do not shift down some gears the pedaling may become so difficult that you will have to get off and walk the bike--not all that bad (it is, after all, still exercise) but most of us would rather be able to keep pedaling (if we had wanted to walk we'd have gone on a hike). As you approach the hill you should try to pick up your speed a bit to help with the initial incline, shift into the middle front sprocket, then, when the pedaling becomes difficult, shift down a gear using the rear sprockets. As soon as the pedaling becomes difficult again, shift down again. Don't wait until the pedaling is very difficult or the shifting will be difficult. Try to anticipate when you will need to shift. If the hill is so steep that you are going to need the smallest front sprocket shift to it before getting to the lowest rear sprocket so the change in revolutions will not be so drastic. This will take a little practice but is not that difficult to master. If, after you've gotten to the lowest gear and the hill is still too steep to ride up, just get off the bike and walk it up--there's nothing wrong with that. Most of the time, however, it will actually be easier and faster to climb the hill riding so it is worth the effort to learn to shift your way to the top. I've read that standing up to pedal doesn't really give you more power but sometimes it just feels better. I have a friend who likes to "attack the hill" by trying to get up it as fast as he can. He says, "It's going to hurt--whether it hurts for a short time or a long time is up to you." That's where the ego gets involved, though, and that doesn't always make for the best decisions. If the hill is too steep or too long and the pedaling is just too difficult, put the ego aside and do what is right for you.

ANECDOTE

In the fall of 1997 my friend, Eric, and I rode from Manitowoc, WI around Michigan's Upper Peninsula to Ludington, MI and took the ferry, the S. S. Badger, across Lake Michigan back to Manitowoc. Michigan Hwy. 2, with wide shoulders and not too much traffic (it would be heavier in the summer, I'm sure) made for a nice, scenic ride across the top of Lake Michigan. At Mackinac Bridge, which connects the U. P. with the rest of the state, we had to get a lift across the bridge from the Bridge Authority as no bicycles are allowed on the bridge, which is approximately five miles long. In preparation for the ride I had contacted the Michigan State Highway Patrol, as I was in law enforcement myself, and had been directed to Trooper Dave Kunzy, who is also a cyclist, and he had given me tips on routes across the area. He told me Hwy. 2 was a safe route and suggested I plan to ride the "Tunnel of Trees" along the eastern shore of Lake Michigan. We took his advice and thoroughly enjoyed the ride which follows Michigan Hwy. 119 from Cross Village, through Good Hart (where we got snacks and a great locally-brewed root beer at the general store/post office), and on to Harbor Springs. The road is on the bluffs overlooking Lake Michigan and on the bright, sunny day several shades of blue could be seen in the lake, reminding us of the Caribbean Sea. The route is called The Tunnel of Trees, as you may have guessed by now, because for fifteen miles or more the road is graced with a canopy of treetops making it look and feel as if you are riding through a tunnel. It was just one of the highlights of this particular trip.

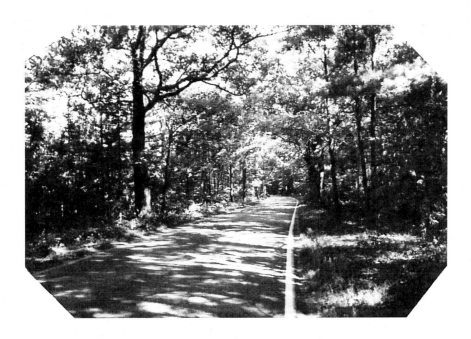

The Tunnel of Trees in Michigan.

Chapter 5
Equipment

Hopefully, after some riding, you've decided to continue to ride the bike rather than leave it hanging in the garage. If so, you may want to think about equipping the bike, and yourself, with things that will make your rides even more pleasant. You don't need all the bells and whistles, and maybe not any of them, but some of them may fit the way you want to ride. It will depend on how you plan to use the bike. If you plan on just riding around the neighborhood for a half-hour at a time you won't need anything else. If, however, you want to take longer rides in varying traffic or scenic conditions and during which weather conditions may change, you may get hungry and thirsty, or want to know how far you've gone (and how far you have to go to get back), there are products that will help you. As you use the bike more you will find out which of these would make the ride better and which ones you really don't need (before buying them).

Helmet and Water Bottle

These were discussed in an earlier chapter. The helmet is a must and the water bottle and holder (or cage) are cheap and very nice to have if you will be on the bike for a longer period of time (more than an hour).

BIKE LOCK

Buying and using a good bike lock may save your bike; your bike store employee can help you find a good one. U-locks are the strongest. Lock the bike, using the frame, even if you are only going to be away from it for a short time. If you'll be away longer try to fit the lock through both the front tire and the frame. Write the bike's serial number down and keep it, you'll need it for a police report if the bike does get stolen.

EYEWEAR

The constant breeze caused by your motion will dry out your eyes so it is a good idea to wear sunglasses or some other kind of eyewear. It isn't that big of a deal on shorter rides but your eyes can get pretty sore over a longer period of time. Eyewear will also protect your eyes from bugs and dust, of course.

PADDED BIKING SHORTS

Biking shorts come with padding in the crotch that really lessens the impact of the bike seat on your seat. Most people think of the tight, spandex shorts when they think of bike shorts but there are other options. For those of us not as comfortable in tight-fitting clothing (I once tried on a pair of spandex shorts and, upon seeing myself in the mirror, thought, "The world's not ready for this.") all-terrain biking shorts come with an inner, tight layer and an outer, looser shell that has pockets. These shorts look more like regular shorts and won't make you feel as if people are staring at you when you go into a restaurant or store. If you like how you look in spandex, however, by all means go for it. It's the padding that is important and either kind of short will make riding more comfortable.

Toe Clips

Don't let the name fool you, toe clips don't actually clip your toes to the pedals. Don't confuse them with the "clip-in" shoes you see more serious riders using which actually do clip into the pedal. Toe clips are small "basket-like" devices that attach to the pedals and into which you slip your feet. Most have straps to allow you to tighten them onto your feet so you can pull up on the pedals, in addition to pushing down, which will improve efficiency and, thus, power. That's great if you are in a race but isn't going to do a lot for the average rider who is probably not going to get used to pulling up on the pedals. Toe clips, however, serve another, more important (in my opinion) purpose, which is to prevent the rider's foot from slipping forward off the pedal. From time-to-time, especially when pedaling hard, your foot can slip forward off the pedal, throwing off your balance and maybe even catching your foot under the front of the pedal. This, obviously, is not something you want to happen. Slipping your foot in and out of the toe clips will take some getting used to--if you don't take your foot out of the device when you come to a stop you will not be able to put the foot on the ground and if you don't put your foot on the ground you will tip over--but once you get used to them you'll find them useful. There are some that come without straps and just keep the foot from going forward that are easier to use. When you first start to use them you have to consciously tell yourself, "Take my foot out." as you approach a stop, but it shouldn't take long before it is second-nature. I use the strapless toe-clips with my hybrid but have clip-in shoes for my road bike. You don't actually need toe clips but you may want to get a set. It depends on how much riding you plan to do.

Clip-Ins

I only put this in to tell readers to <u>not</u> get clip-ins until they have ridden for some time and are very comfortable on the bike. Clip-ins throw a whole new dynamic into it and new riders don't need the added pressure. In this system the shoe clips into the pedal and can only be removed with a twist of the foot. This takes some getting used to as a rider has to anticipate when a stop is imminent (and not all stops are that obvious) and must remember to "unclip" before the stop. If you forget you're clipped in as you approach a stop, by the time you figure out why your leg won't go down it's too late and you'll fall. This can be humorous to watch as it all happens in slow motion. You see the rider come to a stop, wonder why the leg isn't going down, then slowly lean to one side or the other until he or she hits the ground (like Artie Shaw on the tricycle in "Laugh-In" years ago). While this is humorous to watch, it is not funny to the person doing the falling, so keep your laughter to a minimum--once the rider gets untangled from the bike he or she may very well be able to catch you.

Gloves

As you start to ride more you may find your fingers going numb on longer rides. This happens, I believe, from the pressure put on the hands from leaning onto the handlebars. I've been told that this is cumulative, meaning the more it happens the more likely it is to happen again (and become more severe). A pair of biking gloves with padding in the palm and fingers will prevent this. Shaking the arms and hands from time-to-time while riding also helps. The gloves don't have to be expensive--$15 or so should do it. Replace them depending on how much you ride or on the wear. When the padding is worn down, replace the gloves. A pair of gloves lasts me a year.

Computer

An inexpensive computer will tell you your speed, distance traveled for the year, distance traveled for this particular ride, elapsed time, average speed, time of day, and your cholesterol level (okay, I'm kidding about that last one). This is nice to know but not particularly necessary. If you are a "techy" and love your gadgets, remember that you have to read the computer while riding so if you get a complicated one you may end up riding into a parked car while trying to figure out the barometric pressure. A cheap one ($25 or so) will do. "Keep it simple, stupid!" applies here. Get one with just two relatively large buttons that can be easily seen and pushed while riding and a minimum of functions.

Racks and Bags

A rear and or front rack to which bags can be attached is nice. There are many styles of bags that attach to a rack, from a grocery bag-sized bag made for bringing groceries home to saddlebags (panniers) for carrying a week's worth of supplies to a smaller bag that fits onto the rear rack and can carry everything you'll need for a day-long ride. I would suggest a rear rack and bag that attaches to the top of it for most people. That bag will carry a rain jacket or warmer shirt in case the weather changes, snacks, cell phone, car keys, sun screen, etc. There are also handlebar bags that just clip to the handlebars and need no rack but if they are big enough to carry a lot they can also effect steering. Whatever kind of bag fits your needs, it is nice to have a place to carry things on a longer ride. When you buy a bag check how it attaches to the bike. If you have to get down on your hands and knees and wind straps under the rack, then back out and through a holder on the bag, then back under the rack, you're going to be pretty irritated by the time the bag is on (I speak from experience here). You can now get bags that quickly and easily attach to a rack.

Inner Tube/Tire Irons/Pump

It's good to have an inner tube (make sure you get the right size), tire irons (small plastic tools that help get the tire off), and a small pump with you in case of a flat tire. Even if you don't know how to fix the tire you may meet another cyclist who can help you do it (and we love to help). Of course, it's best to learn to change the tire and it really isn't that difficult. A cell phone works even better if you can get in touch with a friend to come and get you.

Mirror

Being able to see traffic behind you increases safety and a mirror allows you to do so without looking over your shoulder (which can cause the rider to veer that way). There are mirrors that mount on the bike helmet but I prefer handlebar mirrors as they are bigger. Mount the mirror on the left side of the bike and get into the habit of checking it often as you ride. If nothing else it will be nice to see the color of the truck that is about to run you over (just kidding).

Bell

I have a bell on each bike that can be rung as I approach pedestrians or other cyclists from behind to let them know I'm approaching. Both bells came with a "rotating dinger" and I always say you can have more fun with a rotating dinger. Of course, a verbal warning works just as well.

Fenders

Plastic, light-weight fenders will help keep water and trail dirt off the back of your shirt and dust from flying up and into your eyes from the front wheel. They aren't necessary but can make you more comfortable. Some racks are solid on top so may take the place of fenders to some extent. Most fenders now are light, quiet plastic, not the large chrome ones of our youth, and don't detract too much from the looks of the bike (at least a hybrid).

Anecdote

There is a sign on a bike trail in northwestern Minnesota that reads "Attn.: Cyclists are advised to wear bright-colored clothing during hunting season." I've always wondered if that's so they can miss us or hit us. I try not to think about it too much. And there's a nature's preserve near my home with a great bike trail I use often. In the fall of the year, as there are too many deer living in the preserve so close to a metropolitan area, the city hires hunters to "cull the herd" with an archery hunt. During those two weekends they put up signs that read, "Caution--Archery Hunt In Progress--Stay on Paved Trails." I always figure I'll just find somewhere else to ride for the weekend.

These two related items remind me of a trip I took at the end of the season one year in southern Minnesota. It was early November (yes, I was pushing the season) and I left Preston riding the Root River Trail to Lanesboro, then on to Houston, Minn., where I stayed the night. As I rode between Preston and Lanesboro on the trail I noticed a large flock of wild turkeys on my right gorging themselves on a harvested cornfield and thought of how lucky I was to see the sight. I then noticed movement on my left and, looking that way, saw several men in camouflage clothing carrying shotguns also watching the flock of turkeys. I put my head down and pedaled as fast as I could and spent the rest of the ride somewhat nervous.

The next day I had ridden to Harmony, Minn. and stopped for a late lunch before the last leg of the trip, about ten or twelve miles back to Preston. As I had been on the bike trail to Preston before, I asked the owner of the café if there were a different route. He suggested that I ride "the ridge," a scenic county road that went above the long valley all the way to Preston, but warned that I would have to take on a long hill to get to the ridge. I took his advice and he was right, the view was worth the climb. As I approached Preston, which is nestled in the valley, the weather was overcast and it was getting dark. As I started my descent back into the valley and caught first sight of the small town its lights were on and it looked like one of those Snow Village displays you see in stores--very quaint and pretty.

It started to rain as I put the bike on my car (which I had left in Preston the day before) and I thought I was lucky to have finished before the rain. I drove home to St. Paul and the next day, when I picked up my local paper, saw that Preston and southeastern Minnesota had gotten thirteen inches of snow overnight. I had been luckier than I had realized.

Chapter 6
Commuting

Years ago, I decided to bicycle the ten miles to work twice a week to use less fuel (polluting less and saving money), get exercise (I seldom wanted to work out after getting home from a day of work), and enjoy the commute more (a good portion of the commute was on very nice trails). As the sedan I was driving then (I now drive a hybrid--and love it) was getting twenty miles per gallon of gas I figured I was saving two gallons of gas a week. It worked so well that in a very short time I was riding four days a week and only taking the car the other day so I could do errands on the way home. I was fortunate that my workplace had a place to store my bike and a locker room where I could shower, although I found that on most days if I rode a little easier to work in the cool of the morning I could get by with just washing up. When I got home at night I had my exercise done for the day and was less tense as I had ridden home through meadows and woods, past lakes, and had listened to birds singing and the wind in the trees rather than having sat in rush-hour traffic listening to roaring trucks and blaring horns.

Commuting can work very well if the situation is right, but if the commute takes you into heavy traffic or is long it may not be worth it. Car-pooling or mass-transit are other alternatives, of course.

Weather will be a factor, also. We've all heard of people who ride to work year-round, even in the northern climes, but that isn't practical for most of us. I've always thought that motorists just don't expect to see bicyclists during the winter months and the snow piled on the shoulders and sometimes on the roads themselves make it difficult for cyclists to give enough room to vehicles. I put the bikes away after the first lasting snowfall.

During the warmer months or in warmer areas, however, commuting by bike may work for you. It takes a bit of organization, however. Depending on your job, you may need a place to shower and change when you get there (I had many jobs over the years in which a shower before work didn't make sense). You will probably need a way to carry your work clothing with you, although you may be able to leave some of the clothing in your work locker, so you'll have to get racks and bags for the bike. I had friends who would had "blue weeks" or "brown weeks" depending on the color of the sport jacket they left in their locker. They changed the jacket once a week and brought the easier to carry clothing each day. You will need, of course, a place to safely store the bike.

Plan a route to and from work that will take you away from traffic as best you can. Some cities have buses with bike racks so you can bus part of the way and most cities have bike trails and less-used roadways that can get you close to where you need to go while keeping you out of heavy traffic. Using them may take you a bit out of your way but will be well worth it if it keeps you out of traffic. Chances are, however, that you are going to have to ride on some busier streets somewhere during the commute. If that is the case don't try to commute until you are comfortable riding in traffic. If you live in a less urban area try to find low-traveled county roads, preferably with good shoulders, to get to work. Remember, a normally low-traffic road may be more busy during "rush hours"--pay attention to the traffic levels as you drive to and from work for several days.

Wherever you live, it is a good idea to scout a route before actually using it to commute. That will allow you to see how long it will take, how far out of the way you will have to go, what obstacles there are to a quick ride, etc. without worrying about getting to work on time.

Commuting will entail getting up earlier and getting home a bit later but the advantages may well outweigh the disadvantages.

You will save money on gas, use less resources, pollute less, get exercise, have time to wake up fully on the way to work, and have time to wind-down on the way home. With a little effort you will probably be able to plan a route that allows you to ride through some nice, relaxing areas in contrast to driving home in tense, rush-hour traffic.

Don't give up on the idea of commuting because it won't always work or there a couple of problems. You can probably overcome the problems with a bit of imagination. Try it once to see if it works. If it does, commit to commuting once or twice a week and you may find, as I did, that you want to do it more often.

ANECDOTE

For several years I followed my son's American Legion baseball team as they traveled around the Midwest playing tournaments. I always took my bike along and rode in the morning as the games were in the late afternoon or evening. One August we were in Fargo, N. D. for a weekend tournament and I drove south to the Sheyenne National Grassland hoping to find a trail to ride. There was no trail but I found some good county-road riding through the prairie. The day started out hot, got hotter, and by noon the temperature was 101 degrees! The road was an east-west road and there was a thirty-mile-per-hour wind from the south so I was getting some evaporation cooling. About an hour into the ride, at an intersection with another county road, I noticed a sign that read "Scenic View--3 Miles" with an arrow pointing south, into the wind. As the countryside was flat prairie I wanted to see what the scenic view could possibly be so I turned into the wind and rode the three miles. The view turned out to be the start of a twenty-five mile hiking trail and was almost worth pedaling into the wind for three miles to see. I turned to go back and thought, "At least riding back will be easy with the wind at my back."

Normally, as you ride you create a breeze from your forward motion. But if you have a tailwind, you have to get up to the speed of the wind moving past you, literally ride faster than the wind, before you feel the breeze from your forward motion. Within minutes of starting the three-mile ride back I realized that with the strong wind directly behind me I could not outride the wind. I was going fast enough that the tailwind was not cooling me but not fast enough to get the breeze from my forward motion. So here I was, riding in 101 degrees and not getting any cooling effect. It felt as though I was riding in a vacuum and have never been so hot. If the ride back to the intersection had been much more than three miles I would not have been able to continue. Once I turned so the wind was a crosswind I was fine, hot but not too hot. That was an interesting phenomenon.

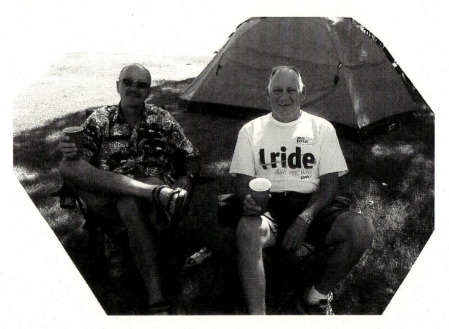

Author and friend, Steve, enjoying the "best part of the day" after a long ride in North Dakota.

Chapter 7
Accidents

Motorcyclists have a saying--"There are two kinds of motorcyclists, those who have had an accident and those who are going to have an accident." The point being if you ride long enough you are going to have an accident. It isn't quite that bad in cycling but you get the point--accidents are always a possibility. A bicycle/motor vehicle accident is, obviously, more serious for the cyclist, so you should be aware while you are riding and do everything you can to lessen your chances of a collision. The best way to avoid accidents is to understand what causes them.

According to the Minnesota Dept. of Transportation the main causes of bicycle/motor vehicle accidents are:

Factors attributed to bicyclists:
Failure to yield right-of-way
Inattention/distraction
Disregard traffic control device
Improper/unsafe lane use

Factors attributed to motorists:
Failure to yield right-of-way
Driver inattention/distraction
Vision obscured

Three of the best ways to avoid accidents are: <u>Be aware! Be aware! Be aware!</u> You and the bike will weigh around 200 to 250 lbs.; a motor vehicle weighs between 5,000 and 50,000 lbs. Not much of a contest. Keep in mind that you and your bike will lose almost every accidental encounter with a motor vehicle and ride accordingly. The motorist risks a dented fender, you are risking your health--and maybe more.

Do everything you can do to stay out of harm's way. Be on the lookout for conditions that will hide your presence from motorists. If you are riding west into a setting sun (or east into a rising sun--although I don't recommend getting up that early), know that a driver may not see you and ride as far to the right as you can. You may even have to consider pulling off to the side of the road to let traffic pass and then find a less busy route home. When approaching a curve or hillcrest, check your mirror to see if any cars are approaching from behind. If so, make sure the drivers see you by weaving back and forth a bit. Try to get around the curve or over the hill soon enough to put enough space between you and the vehicle so the driver will have time to see you and react after cresting the hill or coming around the curve. Remember that many drivers use the shoulder to go around a curve (which means they are going too fast) and may not give you the space they should.

Many bicycle/motor vehicle accidents are caused by cyclist error and the cyclist can avoid them by <u>not causing them.</u> Other accidents could be avoided by just being aware of your surroundings and conditions. A cyclist, like a driver, should always be looking for situations that can cause a problem. Don't assume that the driver of the car at the stop sign sees you. Make eye contact and be ready to swerve or brake if need be. If the roadway is narrow and heavily traveled, find another route. Take care of yourself.

It has been my experience that the more tired I become the more prone I am to make a mistake. I have found myself, at the end of a long ride, shifting up instead of down, forgetting to signal my turns, not paying attention to traffic behind me, and making other minor errors that could cause a major problem. Now, as the day wears on, I keep that fact in mind and, therefore, am more vigilant.

According to the bicycling safety organization Share the Road (www.sharetheroadmn.org) a 1996 study found that cyclists are twice as likely to have an accident riding a multi-use trail and twenty-five times more likely when riding a sidewalk than riding on the road. Therefore, the organization advises riding on a roadway even when adjacent sidewalks and bike trails are available. I would think that the bike trails in the study were trails alongside and crossing roadways and not the long trails going mostly through countryside (although the road crossings on rural trails can be hazardous and should be approached accordingly).

A cyclist should always give a parked car a three foot clearance in order to avoid running into the car door if an occupant of the car suddenly opens the door.

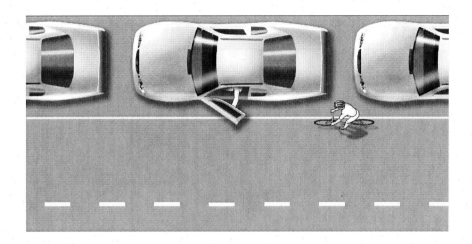

You should always ride in a predictable manner and let motorists know what your intentions are by signaling turns. One of the main causes of accidents listed by the National Highway Transportation Safety Administration is the cyclist swerving to the left without checking traffic or signaling. Other causes listed are the cyclist riding against traffic and cyclists disobeying stop signs.

According to Share the Road fifty percent of crashes occur when the bicyclist and motorist are on crossing or perpendicular paths and three-quarters of these are caused by one or the other not yielding the right-of-way. So it makes sense to be wary as you approach an intersection (street, alley, or driveway). The most serious accidents, however, occur when a motor vehicle overtakes the bicycle from behind, presumably because the speeds are higher in this type of accident.

According to the Bicycle Helmet Safety Institute forty-five to eighty-eight percent of brain injuries from bicycling accidents could be prevented by a bike helmet, so, once again, wear a helmet.

Now that I have frightened you out of riding your bike anywhere but your garage let me say that things aren't as bad as this chapter may have made them sound. With awareness, common sense, and a healthy respect for motor vehicles you can keep yourself pretty well out of harm's way. I once rode with someone for the first time and after an hour told him that if he were my child I would spank him and send him home (relax, I would never really spank a child; I would write a strongly-worded letter expressing my disappointment followed by an apology for being too stern). My friend ran stop signs, rode on the wrong side (even on major highways), made turns without signaling, and made U-turns without thinking how he was affecting other traffic. I was embarrassed (as his riding reflected badly on me, too), and, frankly, concerned for his safety. He was riding in a way that was unsafe for him and discourteous to others on the roadway.

I have found that it is safer for the cyclist to ride as if he or she is a motor vehicle. Imagine yourself riding a motorcycle--you wouldn't cut between cars, ride on the wrong side of the road, or run stop signs and red lights on a motorcycle.

A little courtesy will go along way, too. Most of us drive a good deal and we don't want someone turning in front of us without signaling, or running stop signs in front of us, or taking up the driving lane when there is a perfectly good shoulder on which to ride, etc. Ride your bicycle as you would want someone to ride in front of you.

Don't be afraid to ride on roadways, but keep in mind that wherever you ride there is a chance of an accident (a recent news item told of a man who was riding a wilderness mountain biking trail and ran into a bear) and take the steps to lower the risks.

ANECDOTE

There came a day when I knew I'd been riding too much and was a bit too interested in cycling. I was on a 70-mile ride from my house on a route that would take me through the small village of Afton, Minn. and up a series of steep hills to Afton State Park, then on to Red Wing, Minn. As I was leaving Afton, about to tackle the hills, I noticed, standing alongside her bike on the side of the road ahead, a shapely young lady. She was wearing one of those tight-fitting one-piece biking outfits that I find very attractive and slathering herself with suntan lotion. Her bicycle was a brand new, expensive, high-tech bike with the "floating seat" (one that is not attached to a vertical bar so the rider won't feel the bumps so much). As I passed her and said, "Hi," I looked her way and, honestly, the first thing that popped into my mind was, "What a nice bike!" Now, I have as much appreciation for an attractive lady as the next guy (inherited from my father who used to tell my mom that he kept his eyes open while kissing her in case a pretty lady walked past) so I was appalled that the first thought in my mind was of the bike. The second thought, by the way, was that I wanted to get up the hills before she finished putting on the lotion because I knew she would pass me on the hills otherwise. Sure enough, about halfway up the series of hills she breezed by me with a cheery, "Hi. Nice day, huh?" so quickly that she probably didn't hear my gasping reply.

Chapter 8
More Comfortable Riding

There are several things a rider can do to make riding more comfortable.

A Good Fit

First of all, getting a good fit to the bike will help you avoid many problems with comfort. That's where a reputable bike shop comes in handy. A good bike shop will fit you with the right bike and make sure the pedals, handlebars, and seat are set in the proper spots in conjunction with your body. This isn't a long, scientific process--they will be able to do it just by "eyeballing" things. If you are just going to use the old bike it would be a good idea to go into the bike shop you are going to use for a tune-up or repairs and ask the person there to see how you fit the bike and make any necessary adjustments. This might cost you a little but will be well worth it in the long run. Handlebars that are set too low can cause hand and arm numbness and a seat set even slightly too high or low can cause knee pain. If you decide to ride longer rides than just around the neighborhood I recommend getting a "fitting."

Hands and Arms

Over the course of a long ride the cyclist's hands, fingers, and perhaps even arms may become numb and/or sore from the constant pressure on the palms. Padded cycling gloves, as I already pointed out, will help alleviate this, as will shaking the hands and arms periodically and holding the arms, one at a time, of course, above the head for a short time. Just changing positions on the handlebars will help, also. A set of bar-end handlebars, extensions of the regular handlebars, will give the rider a different angle at which to hold the bars and, thus, change the pressure points on the hands giving the palms a respite. I wouldn't advise "aero-bars," the bars that extend forward from the regular bars and allow the rider to lean far forward and rest on the arms, for new riders as the position changes the dynamics of balance and steering and takes some getting used to.

SHOCK ABSORBERS

Some bikes come with built-in shock absorbers but these add weight and cost to the bike. Fortunately, the human body also comes with built-in shock absorbers, called "legs," and they don't add weight or cost. If you see a bump or hole in the road coming, push yourself up slightly to get your rear end off the seat and flex your legs as you hit the bump. Don't stand up, just lift your body a fraction and bend your legs so the legs will soften the blow.

SAVE YOUR BUNS

At some point on a longer ride your bottom is going to get sore and/or numb. When people ask me if it ever gets to the point that I don't get sore and numb back there I tell them it doesn't, I just get used to being sore. It helps if you stand up and let the blood run back into that area. Obviously, you have to wait until it is safe to stand up--not going around a curve or downhill. Standing up once in a while also lets your legs stretch out a bit. Frequently changing position, even slightly, on the saddle will help limit soreness and numbness. Riding "light on the saddle" will also help. Push up slightly with your legs so your buttocks isn't taking all of the pressure.

On long rides chafing on the buttocks and crotch (sorry to be so blunt) can sometimes be a problem. There are lotion products, found in bike stores, made specifically to prevent or ease chafing. If you forget to use them and chafing occurs these products will relieve the area and prevent further chafing (better late than never).

FOOD AND WATER

It's imperative that you have water with you on a longer ride so you can stay hydrated which helps ward off cramps as well as just being good for you. If you think you'll be getting hungry while on the ride bring food with you or just stop at a convenience store to get something. On a longer ride you should drink before you get thirsty and eat before you get hungry so you don't get behind on energy. Some cyclists insist on eating high- protein bars specially made for energy replacement but I've found that Dairy Queens or their equivalents carry delicious energy foods that you don't have to choke down with water.

CLOTHING

This has been covered earlier but wear comfortable clothing that is not going to chafe and will keep you warm enough in cool weather and cool enough in warm weather. Layering will help accomplish this. If you have a bag attached to the bike, use it to store a light jacket or shirt. If you don't have a bag and want to take off the top layer, tie it around your waist.

SUN PROTECTION

Obviously, use sun screen and sunglasses when appropriate and on longer rides use lip balm. I hate the feel of lip balm, but not as much as I hate the feel of chapped lips.

ANECDOTE

In 1995 My friend, Eric, with whom I have had many pleasant week-long bike rides, and I did a ride in Upstate New York and Vermont (see Ch. 1). We started in Burlington, Vt., rode around Lake Champlain with a side trip through part of the Adirondack Mountains to Lake Placid, and back to Burlington. One day, after a long day of riding through the mountains when arrived in Port Henry, NY with plans to make it to Vermont by late afternoon. As we rode south out of Port Henry we saw a road sign that read, "Bridge to Vermont--8 Miles." We looked east across a narrow part of the lake and could see a bridge that at least appeared to be within a half-mile. As we were tired, hot, and worn out from the trip through the mountains I said, "That better not be the bridge to Vermont." We rode four miles south to an adjoining road that went northeast and saw another sign reading, "Bridge to Vermont--4 Miles." Sure enough, the bridge that had seemed so close in Port Henry was, indeed, the bridge to Vermont. We had to ride eight miles to cover what couldn't have been more than a mile across the water!

Another fifteen miles or so brought us to the very beautiful, exclusive Basin Harbor Club on the shore of Lake Champlain. As we stood in line at the registration desk Eric, who is somewhat, shall we say, frugal, turned to me and said, "If it's under $300 we're taking it!" The room was only $150 and we spent a pleasant night at the resort. Lake Champlain, despite being cold, made for a wonderfully refreshing dip after the hard, hot day of riding.

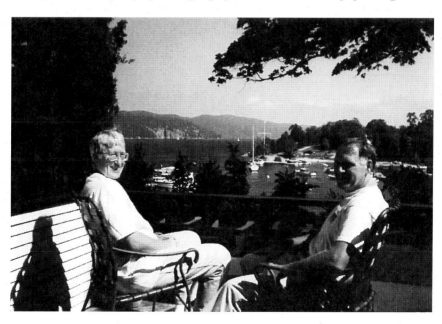

Author and his friend, Eric, relaxing at The Basin Harbor Club.

Chapter 9
More Serious Riding

After riding the bike for a while you may come to one of several conclusions. You may decide that the bike will best serve you by hanging out of the way on the garage wall. If so, that's fine; at least you gave it a shot and now know it just isn't for you. This is the reason you (hopefully) took my advice and didn't buy the expensive bike. Now you can stop saying, "Someday I'm going to…." and start saying, "I tried that but didn't particularly like it."

You may also decide biking around the neighborhood is all the riding you need to do right now and leave open the possibility of longer rides for sometime in the future.

Or you may decide riding bike is really great and want to take the next step--more serious riding. More serious riding encompasses several aspects of cycling including the "way" you ride, riding in imperfect weather, traffic, and length of ride.

The Way You Ride

What does this mean? As you ride around the neighborhood the streets are mostly quiet; traffic is light and motor vehicle speeds are low. The rider often has nowhere in particular to go and is just meandering in a small radius around home on streets with few lane markings. There aren't many decisions to be made. He should be alert, obey all traffic laws, and generally be aware of his surroundings.

As the cyclist branches out, however, things become more complicated. Traffic will be heavier and faster, there will be more lanes and traffic signs, and the cyclist's speed will be greater. All this adds up to more decisions to be made and more import to those decisions. When you start "cycling" as compared to "bike riding" you are going to have to become even more alert and even a bit wary, constantly watching for situations that could lead you into trouble. You should get into a "self-defense mindset" and keep safety in your mind at all times. This may lessen your enjoyment somewhat but if being wary helps you avoid an accident it will be well worth it. As you're approaching a driveway take a quick look to see if there are trees, bushes, or other obstructions that may hide your presence from a driver leaving the drive. As you approach a curve on the bike trail be aware that there may be something (a dog, a person, a deer) on the trail that you may not be able to see until you get around the curve (at which time it may be too late to stop). I could give a thousand scenarios but you get the idea. Always be looking for things that might cause you problems and do something to lessen the risks. Check your mirror often. Remember that a cyclist is in a very vulnerable position and must constantly be thinking about safety. Don't get into the "I'm the only one in the world." mode. You are not the only one out there and others' actions will affect you, just as your actions will affect others.

CYCLING FOR EXERCISE

Cycling is an excellent, low-impact exercise; it burns calories, strengthens the cardiovascular system, builds muscles and endurance, and improves overall fitness. And you don't have to drive to the club to do it; you can start right from your garage. Plan out a route that won't take you through too much traffic and doesn't have too many stop signs and turns so you can keep a steady pace. You can get a "fancy-dancy" heart monitor if you wish but just the fact that you're breathing hard should be a good indication of heart rate. Check with your physician, of course, if you are unsure you are healthy enough to ride more strenuously. Start with a short distance and lengthen it and/or ride it faster as you become more fit. Find routes with hills, which will challenge you more; then, after a while, find larger hills. Use common sense, you know your body better than anyone else. You don't have to ride long distances to get exercise.

Imperfect Weather

There will be times when you want to ride even when the weather is not perfect, or, you are on a longer ride and the weather changes, leaving you riding home in a driving rain. I tell people that I <u>can</u> ride in all sorts of bad weather but I seldom <u>choose</u> to do so. I ride for pleasure and riding in a thunderstorm is neither fun nor smart. On the other hand, I'm not going to give up a longer ride because of the possibility of showers later in the day.

Rain

You can ride in a light rain all day if you have to. It won't be as pleasant but it shouldn't keep you from getting home on the bike. A brightly-colored rain slicker will help a bit but you might as well face the fact that you're going to get wet. Like my mom used to say, "You won't melt." Keep in mind you won't be as visible to motorists. Riding through a lightening storm on a piece of metal, however, is just downright foolish. If you're stuck in a thunderstorm pull over and find shelter (<u>not</u> under a tree) until the storm passes or you can get home some other way.

Moisture, even in warm weather, can make the surface slippery--this is especially true on fallen leaves.

Wind

Riding into a stiff wind can be daunting. I'd rather have hills than a headwind because you never get to the top of the wind and you can't coast down the other side. Just like you wouldn't paddle a canoe downstream first, try to plan your ride so you are riding into the wind during the first half when you are fresher (and riding home with the wind at your back can be a real pleasure). If you have to ride into the wind to get where you are going try to alternate the route a bit to give yourself a respite, however brief, from the battle. There will be times, however, when you just have to downshift, put your head down, and "plod along" one stroke at a time. If you are riding with a friend, drafting (see below) will help.

Tornadoes

Just seeing if you're paying attention.

Cold Weather

Cold weather doesn't have to stop you from riding, you just have to dress appropriately. There are a lot of cycling cold-weather clothing items you can buy but I'll bet you have things that will work stored in your closet. I find that the parts of my body that are most difficult to keep warm are my fingers and my toes so I have neoprene boots to go over my shoes and good gloves.

Snow

Those of us in the northern climes should put the bikes away for the season after the first lasting snow and take out the skis. Drivers don't expect to see cyclists out in winter weather and it is difficult to move out of the flow of traffic when there are snow banks narrowing the traffic lanes. If you absolutely insist on riding throughout the winter watch for my next book, "Cycling for the Overly-Zealous."

Drafting

If you are riding on a windy day with a friend or friends try "drafting" one another. As a rider rides through the wind, she produces a slight "pocket of stillness" in her wake or her side opposite the wind. If another rider can fit into this pocket, he will be protected from the wind and not have to pedal as hard. This maneuver is called "drafting" and takes a bit of concentration as it involves riding in close single file--a two foot gap between tires will do the trick and still be fairly safe. The more people in the line the easier it is for the last rider and the more rest for all riders as each takes a turn in the front. The lead rider should stay in front for only a short time, then move to the rear of the line, letting the next rider in line take the lead. This will give each rider a rest, keeping all of them fresher. If the rider in front stays too long he will tire and may have trouble keeping up when it is his turn to ride in back. If a rider is markedly stronger than the others she may want to stay in front longer but shouldn't take on too much. When the rider in front wants to rest she signals her intent, moves slightly to the left, lets the line pass her, then pulls into the last spot. The dynamics of the group can be figured out as the riders go along and, with a bit of practice, the transition can be done smoothly and without missing a beat. You don't need a long line, though, drafting can be quite effective with just two riders.

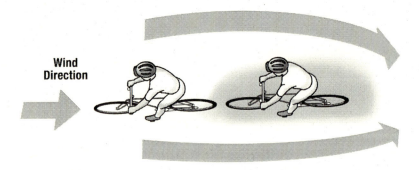

Again, drafting takes a good bit of concentration as the riders' tires are very close to each other and one rider slowing or swerving suddenly can upset the others. I never draft, at least closely, with others if I haven't ridden with them long enough to know how they ride. When riders I don't know try to draft me I wave them by. Drafting with someone takes a certain level of trust and knowledge of their riding style and I can't have either of these if I haven't ridden with a person. Some riders forget that if they are going to be in the back to enjoy the benefits of drafting they should also ride point now-and-again to do their share of the work.

Drafting works well even when the wind isn't a direct headwind. If the wind is from the front and left the riders can line up in an "echelon" or wing formation from left to right with each rider behind and to the right of the lead rider. Each rider can settle into the space that has the least wind resistance. This, of course, takes up more room on the road and will not be safe or practical in many cases but, in the right set of circumstances or with just two riders, can work quite nicely.

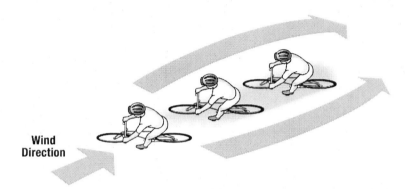

COMMUNICATING

While riding with others it is a good idea to communicate with each other using signals of some sort, as talking may be impractical at times. If you are in the lead and have to go around broken glass, debris, or a hole you should point to it as you go by to let those behind you know something is there. If you are on a street and see a parked car ahead with an occupant who may open the door, point at the car and shout, "Car door!" This may also alert the occupant of the car to your presence.

Bicycles are quiet so you may want to make some kind of noise to alert motorists, pedestrians, or other cyclists to your approach. This is where the bell will come in handy but if you don't have one just start talking to the person.

Taking the Lane

While cyclists should ride as far to the right of a roadway as they can to help the flow of traffic, there are times when it is advisable to "take the lane" by moving to the center of the lane to discourage motorists from passing. When the lane narrows to a point that a passing vehicle will force you too close to a guard rail or other obstruction, or on a four lane street with lanes so narrow that a vehicle using the inside lane to pass a vehicle in the outside lane will come too close to you for safety, riding in the middle of your lane may be the safest thing to do. This lets motorists know there isn't room to pass safely and doesn't "tempt" the impatient ones to try. Obviously, a cyclist won't want to take the lane for any length of time, just long enough to safely get across the bridge or until the lane widens. Some motorists will misunderstand and become angry but using the technique in the right situation is safer for the cyclist. Don't feel bad about it, you do have a right to the lane. Do get out of the way as soon as you can, however, out of courtesy to motorists (even the angry, impatient ones--or, should I say, especially the angry, impatient ones).

Turn Lanes

In Share the Road MN's article *Rules of the Road* they write, "According to the concept of *Effective Cycling* developed by John Forester, 'Cyclists fare best when they act and are treated as drivers of vehicles.'" I have found this to be true, although some of it depends on motorists, of course. Too many drivers still think that anything that doesn't have a "hemi" should stay on the sidewalk.

One Sunday afternoon I was riding a busy county road approaching a four-way stop at which I would have to make a left turn. I signaled my move to the left-turn lane and moved up behind a line of cars taking turns at the sign. I moved up with each car and when it became my turn at the sign I yielded to the cars at the cross street, then turned left. As I made the turn a car turned left from the cross street getting close to me in the process and the passenger shouted, "You're not a !★^#+★! car, you know!" I had done everything right and the motorist was still angry at me.

Turns can be tricky on busy roadways. The right turn should be easy enough, but if an impatient motorist tries to get around the cyclist while she is in the lane, even this turn can become hazardous. This might be a good time to take the lane.

Left turns are trickier, especially on busier roads. If there is no turn lane, the cyclist has to be very careful that traffic from behind is going to notice her in the left side of the lane (especially if she has to wait for oncoming traffic to clear). Most motorists don't expect to see a slow-moving, small vehicle in the faster part of the lane. Check traffic behind you and make sure you have time to make the turn before faster-moving traffic overtakes you, even if you have to pull to the side and wait for a moment. If there is a left-turn lane, I signal my move across the lane in which I'm riding, then to the left-turn lane, taking the lane so a motorist doesn't try to move alongside me. If there is a traffic signal and you get stopped at the red light, be ready to move as soon as it turns green so you don't hold up traffic. You can probably accelerate through the turn almost as fast as motorists do so you won't hold them up long, if at all. Move to the right as soon as possible after the turn.

If there are two or more of you, position yourselves as if you were in a car--one person in the driver's seat, one in the passenger's seat, and two in the back seats. Then turn in conjunction with each other. It's a fairly easy maneuver and avoids a long, single file line that holds traffic up longer.

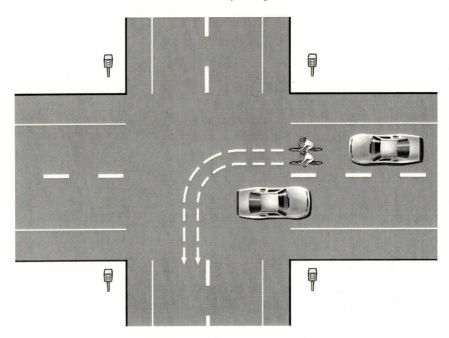

Night Riding

I don't recommend it but if you ride in the dark you need a white light to the front, and a red light and reflectors to the rear. Light-colored, reflective clothing is also a must.

Longer Rides

As you get more into cycling you may want to try your hand (or legs) at longer rides. You can do this on your own, of course, but many organizations sponsor rides. The Multiple Sclerosis Society puts on numerous rides of 50 miles (one day), 150 miles (two days), and 300 miles (five days) and does a very good job of taking care of the participants. Participants are asked to raise donations and a lot of money is raised for a good cause. There are also many day-long and week-long bike rides put on by various organizations that just charge a set fee. If the ride is more than a day the organizer hauls your luggage for you, so all you have to do is ride the bike. Most also have "sag-wagons," so if you tire out or bad weather hits, you can get a lift to the end of that day's ride, food and water stops, and a bike shop mechanic for repairs on the road. These offer a great way to try out a longer ride--you don't have to plan a route, decide where you'll be staying and eating, or worry about breakdowns. All you have to do is ride.

If you decide to give a longer ride a try make sure to build up to longer distances. Riding sixty to eighty miles two, four, or five days in a row takes a little training. Some of the organizations have training schedules they will share but you can probably figure it out on your own. I've been told, and this seems to be about right through my experience, that a cyclist can, over a day, go three times the length she is comfortable riding on her average ride.

ANECDOTE

In 2002 three friends and I rode the KATY Trail State Park, a 225-mile long bike trail across Missouri from St. Charles to Clinton. We stayed the first night in Hermann, Mo., which is across the Missouri River from the KATY, and as we left town to get to the trail, we had to cross the Hermann bridge, a narrow, two-lane structure with no shoulder. To avoid being squeezed against the guard rail by a motorist as we crossed we took the lane, two abreast, and rode as fast as we could to get across without holding up traffic any more than necessary. We crossed the bridge three times that week and each time a vehicle (once a school bus and twice a car) came up behind us, slowed, put its emergency flashers on, and patiently followed us to the other side. The drivers did not show any impatience or anger towards us and we really appreciated the break.

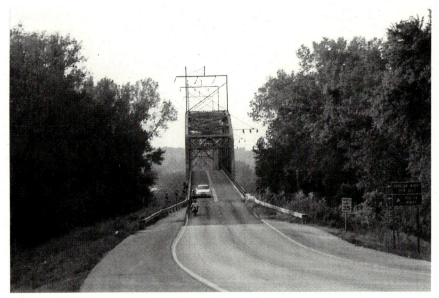

The bridge in Hermann, Missouri--a good place to "take the lane."

Ironically, after having crossed the bridge on our way back into town one evening, we were making our way to our motel along the main street and had to cross a very small, narrow bridge. We rode single-file across it, as it was so short, and as we did a motorist passed us, leaving just inches of clearance. We had done just fine on the long bridge but had almost been done in by the short one.

Chapter 10
Why Cyclists "Do That"

If you ride for any length of time you will eventually be asked, when others learn that you have taken up cycling, "Why do cyclists do that?" about various aspects of riding. Often the word "cyclists" will be accompanied by a colorful descriptor--but let's not get into that. When someone complains about cyclists taking up road space I will ask them to think honestly about how often they have been inconvenienced by a cyclist. I do a good share of driving and can count on one hand the number of times I have been inconvenienced by a cyclist in the past ten years (having to slow down a bit doesn't count). Below are some of the questions I have been asked and my explanations. You're welcome to use them if you end up being cornered some day.

Using the Road

Why do cyclists ride on the roadway when there is an adjacent sidewalk or bike trail? First, I remind the person that cyclists have the right to ride in the roadway whether or not there is a bike trail or sidewalk. I then explain that cyclists are not supposed to ride on sidewalks and many municipalities make it illegal to do so.

As for the bike trails, which are actually multi-use trails, there are many reasons to not use them. In an urban area the cyclist will have to maneuver around people out for a stroll (some of them walking dogs), kids on tricycles, roller-bladers, and other users. Intersections and driveways constitute a hazard as many motorists drive through the trail with nary a glance. Intersections cause another problem-- the trail bed is usually a bit above the street and at each intersection the cyclist has to go over the bumpy transition from the trail to the street and back to the trail. That "ka-thunk, ka-thunk" is hard on the cycle, cycle tires, and cyclist and can cause major veering and lurching. And if a motor vehicle is turning onto or off the cross street a bicycle on the sidewalk or trail causes much more confusion than one riding in the traffic lane.

According to Share The Road a 1996 study showed that bicyclists are <u>twenty-five times</u> more likely to have an accident when riding on a sidewalk than riding on a major street--even one that neither has a designated bike lane nor is designated as a bike route. And bicyclists are twice as likely to have an accident on a multi-use trail than on an unmarked street. So, not only is it safer for cyclists to ride on the road, it's <u>much</u> safer.

SHOULDERS

Why do you ride on the left side of the shoulder, which is closer to the driving lane, instead of on the far right? Shoulders tend to collect debris (broken glass, 2x4's, dead raccoons, etc.) that get pushed farther to the right as traffic goes by at high speeds. There is often more debris on the right side of the shoulder than on the left, much of which (glass, nails) can be seen by the cyclist but not the motorist. Riding closer to the driving lane helps a rider avoid not only the debris but also a sudden swerve around the debris that may "spook" a motorist.

LANE USE

Why do cyclists ride in the middle of the lane instead of getting out of the way? See "Taking the Lane" in Chapter 9.

Jerks on Bikes

I'm sometimes asked why a cyclist would ride down the middle of the lane and not allow traffic the chance to pass even when there is plenty of room to move over. Is that person a jerk? Yes, that person is a jerk, and chances are that person is a jerk while driving a car, too. Wouldn't you rather have that person operating a bike?

Disobeying Traffic Laws

When someone complains about cyclists who run stop signs and red lights or disobey other traffic laws I agree with them that cyclists should obey all traffic laws and tell them it annoys me, also, whether I'm on my bike or in my car. There are many cycling organizations out there and the ones I have had occasion to check out all heavily emphasize obeying traffic laws.

Anecdote

Here are three examples of how cyclists' actions affect motorists and how motorists react:

I was riding a somewhat busy county road one day and watched as a cyclist about a half-block ahead of me, who apparently was still getting used to his clip-in shoes, was forced to come to a quick stop and, being unable to get his shoe detached from the pedal in time, tipped over on the shoulder. To make matters worse, his fall was to the left, thus taking him closer to the driving lane. A motorist passing the cyclist in that lane, who had time to react but did not move over an inch, honked his horn at the cyclist--as if he had fallen on purpose. I wonder if that motorist eventually asked some cyclist he met at a party, "Why do you cyclists fall over in the street?"

While participating in a small organized bike ride on city streets I was in the middle of the pack, not close to any other riders at the time, when a car went past me going the other direction. As the car passed the driver leaned out the window and shouted, "There's a stop sign up there, !#*%#*!" I looked ahead and saw a stop sign about a block up and realized the driver was angry at a cyclist ahead of me who had run the stop sign and he was taking his wrath out on me. Although I had not disobeyed the stop sign, he had seen another cyclist run it, assumed I was also going to run it and, therefore, considered me an !#*%#*.

While riding my exercise route close to home I came to a stop sign at which I would have to turn left so I checked traffic, signaled my turn, moved into the lane, and stopped at the sign. A motorist pulled alongside me on the right, rolled down her window, and said, "Thank you for signaling and stopping at the sign. I wish more cyclists would do that." I assured her I also wished more cyclists would do that and we both drove away feeling better about ourselves and each other.

Chapter 11
How Motorists Can Help Cyclists

There are numerous things motorists can do to help cyclists out and to make things less confusing for all concerned. As most of us drive motor vehicles often, it is good for us to keep these points in mind as we drive. Feel free to pass them on to your non-cycling friends, although it will be better to wait until you are asked to do so.

First, let me say that not everyone riding a bicycle is a "cyclist." Youths riding to the park or the fishing hole, the guy riding his kid's bike to the convenience store for cigarettes (like in the anti-smoking spot on TV--no offense, smoke 'em if you got 'em boys, just don't blow it my way), etc. are people on bicycles, not cyclists. Kids are notorious for thinking they are invincible and thus riding however they wish--on the wrong side of the road, running stop lights, weaving down the middle of the road. They shouldn't do those things but kids will be kids so watch out for them and don't get too angry (unless they're your kids). Adults forced into riding for a short distance by various circumstances are probably just ignorant of how to ride properly (obviously, they haven't read this book). Don't hold their actions against those of us who do ride properly.

I have been asked many times at a party or other gathering, when people hear that I am an avid cyclist, "What's wrong with you people?" They then go on to tell me about how they had to slow down for a pack of cyclists, or their wife saw a cyclist run a stop sign, or some cyclist did some other horrendous deed that made the slighted party late for work, church, the big party, whatever. It always amazes me how the same person who thinks nothing of driving twenty miles-per-hour over the speed limit a car-length behind the car ahead while talking on the cell phone and drinking a cup of coffee will get all bent out of shape if a cyclist doesn't make a full and complete stop (including putting the foot down) at a stop sign in the middle of nowhere! Puleeeze! Have you seen some of the cars slowing for stop signs or turning right on red after slowing just enough to keep all four tires on the ground? I don't think the cyclist on the 25-lb. bike is even close to the biggest problem out there. That having been said, cyclists should obey all traffic laws. Before whining about how they had to ease off their accelerator for an instant drivers should remember that most cyclists drive cars, too, and know just how easy it is to slow down for a second, then speed back up. They're not fooling us with all the wailing and gnashing of teeth. Besides, most people drive too fast, anyway, and slowing down once-in-a-while wouldn't hurt. Now, before drivers turn away in disgust, let me say that we cyclists also realize we can be annoying at times and most of us (the ones without death wishes) do empathize and try to do things to minimize the annoyance factor. Below I list things drivers can do to help cyclists.

SHARE THE ROAD

According to the Minnesota Department Of Transportation bicycles are legal vehicles on all Minnesota roads, except controlled-access highways, and have all the rights and responsibilities as motor vehicles, including the right to operate in a traffic lane. Bicyclists should ride on the road. Motorists must at all times maintain a three-foot clearance when passing a bicyclist. When a motorist is overtaking a bicycle, the bicyclist has the right of way. Bicyclists and motorists must yield the right-of-way to each other equally.

TREAT BICYCLES AS VEHICLES

It is safer for all concerned if driver's treat bicycles as vehicles. You wouldn't stop in traffic and wave an oncoming driver signaling a left turn to turn in front of you, don't do it to a cyclist. While we appreciate it when you treat us so nicely, sometimes it puts us in a bad spot.

OPENING THE CAR DOOR

When you park on a street it's a good idea to check your sideview mirror for an approaching cyclist before opening the door. It's important for the cyclist, of course, but also important for you. My bike and I together weigh just over 200 lbs. (summer weight) and if I hit your open car door at speed there will probably be some damage to the door, too.

SIGNAL YOUR TURNS

Just as it helps drivers when a cyclist or another driver signals a turn, it helps a cyclist when the driver signals. If I know which way you want to go I can usually get out of your way or make it easier for you. If I come upon a right-turn lane but do not plan to turn and I see a car behind me signaling a right turn, I will move as close as I can to the driving lane to allow the car to go past me in the turn lane (if there is enough room to do so safely).

TURNS

When turning left, check for oncoming cyclists. When turning right, yield to cyclists in the lane; don't pass them and then turn abruptly in front of them. Cyclists can reach speeds of 30 m.p.h. or more and speeds of 15 to 25 m.p.h. are common.

HONKING YOUR HORN

If you want to alert a cyclist of your approach (not a bad idea) give a "toot" or two on the horn from afar, don't wait until you are right behind the bike to do it. And if you are one of those people who lay on the horn as you pass just to let us know you have really been put out by our presence on "your" road, I can only assume this paragraph will do no good even if you find someone to read it to you.

Don't Drive on the Shoulder

In Minnesota and, I believe most other states, driving on the shoulder is prohibited at all times. Passing on the shoulder or in the right-turn lane is illegal even if someone is turning left in front of you! One of the few things a cyclist can legally do that a driver can't is operate on the shoulder. If a cyclist or pedestrian is on the shoulder when a driver "blasts" around a left-turning vehicle the results will be disastrous. And if you have to use the shoulder as you drive around a curve you are driving too fast or just being lazy. Again, if a cyclist or pedestrian is on the shoulder just around the curve (especially a kid riding on the wrong side of the road), the result could be a tragedy.

Passing

Passing a cyclist can sometimes be tricky, especially with oncoming traffic, around a curve, or cresting a hill. Remember that slowing down and waiting for a safe opportunity is always an option and won't really cause you that much of a delay. Give the cyclist as much room as you can safely give. Minnesota state law states drivers must give cyclists a three-foot space when passing. There usually is enough room to pass a cyclist without driving into the oncoming lane (if the cyclist is doing his part and riding as far right as practicable). I've had drivers come within inches of me when there was plenty of room for them to move over. Remember that, just like in driving, things happen that can make cyclists veer unexpectedly or even knock us into the lane of traffic through no fault of our own so any space you can give us is appreciated.

Calm Down!

One of my favorite bumper stickers was on the back of St. Paul Police squad cars. It said, simply, "**Calm Down!**" That's a good message all around but especially when approaching a cyclist. Remember that the cyclist or even the pack of cyclists in front of you isn't <u>really</u> going to cause you that much inconvenience. We are just trying to get to or from work, get exercise, or have a pleasant outing. Most of us are pretty good folks and, if you got to know us, you'd probably like us.

Anecdote

In late September of 1999 Eric and I, along with our friend, Dave, drove to the Black Hills of South Dakota to ride the George S. Mickelson Trail, a 114-mile bike trail from Deadwood on the north to Edgemont on the south. We rode it round trip so it was a 228-mile ride, plus a couple of side trips. As the weather in the Black Hills was in the 80's we brought cool-weather clothing (just in case) but left the warmer riding clothes at home--a decision we would regret.

We stopped at Interior, S. D., on the way and had a great day of riding through the fantastic spires and gulches of Bad Lands National Park, then drove on to Hill City, S. D. We awoke the next day to find an inch of snow on the trail and temperatures in the 30's. Fortunately, the cool-weather clothing we had with us retained our body heat, keeping our core bodies fairly warm, but our shoes and gloves were woefully inadequate. We ended up wearing socks over our hands and duct-taping plastic bags over the socks and over our shoes in a feeble attempt to block the wind chill effect. We made for a pretty spiffy-looking group when we stopped for lunch at The Moonshine Gulch Saloon in Rochford (pop. 25). The week after our ride the temperatures in the Black Hills were in the 80's again. It had been just bad timing, and a general lack of preparedness, on our part.

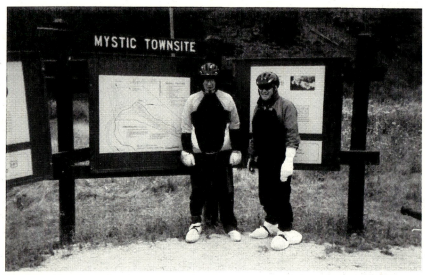
High fashion on the George Mickelson Trail in South Dakota

Chapter 12
The Love of Cycling

By now you have probably figured out that I really love to bicycle. I have gone on many bike rides throughout the United States and one ride in Holland. When I travel by car I take my bike along and stop at interesting places along the way, using the bike to see them up close, then use it at my destination to get exercise and see the area. Most metropolitan areas now have bike trails (maps of which can be found in the local Yellow Pages) and less-populated areas usually have county roads that provide good, safe riding. I go on at least two week-long bike rides a year, as well as two- or three-day overnight rides, and many day-long rides on state trails and on roadways around my house. None of this would have happened if I hadn't taken that first five-mile bike ride.

As well as being an excellent form of exercise, there is something about cycling that gives the rider a sense of "freedom," of being able to go where you want (within reason, of course) at your own pace, and in your own good time. It helps us slow down a bit and get away from our otherwise hectic lives and schedules. I've always thought that I do my best thinking while cycling. A week-long bike ride can be relaxing as we leave the ordinary tasks and worries behind us and all we have to do, especially in an organized event, is ride. Cycling allows us to see the countryside or cityscape at a speed that lets us appreciate what we are seeing. It also gives us more range than walking or running so we can cover more territory.

Riding a bicycle can be a real treat to the senses.

Sights

Seeing wildlife up close is one of the treats of bike riding. Deer seem to think a bike rider is just another animal and, as long as the rider is quiet and doesn't make sharp, sudden movements, will allow a cyclist to coast within feet of them. Once the cyclist stops and puts a foot down, though, the deer will run off. Whatever wild life you have in your area, you will be able to get closer to it on a bike than on foot or in a car. In Minnesota and Wisconsin I have seen eagles, wild turkeys, ospreys, deer, black bear (once a bit too closely), wolves, red and golden fox, turtles, and assorted smaller animals.

In North Dakota I rode past prairie dog villages, heard the prairie dogs whistle warnings of my approach to each other, and watched them duck into their holes (and come back out after I passed). I saw wild horses and antelope in the distance and rode past (again, a bit too closely for comfort) bison grazing on the prairie.

Indigo buntings, bluebirds, orioles, gold finches, wrens, and other small birds add to the enjoyment. Once, riding across Wisconsin on a county road, Eric and I noticed red-wing blackbirds, that build nests in the weedy ditches alongside roads, were keeping an eye on us. As we rode past an area a blackbird would fly out of the ditch and go to the top of the nearest telephone pole, appearing to watch us and, as we rode on, would fly to the next pole, then, keeping up with our progress, to the next pole. At that point the blackbird would fly back toward where she had first started to follow us and a different blackbird would pick us up, "escorting" us for three telephone poles. Their "territory," the area over which they seemed to be watching, appeared to be the length between three telephone poles. This went on for the better part of the morning.

While bike trails can be scenic at times, too often the rider is surrounded by trees and shrubs and cannot see beyond the wall of vegetation. County roads offer vistas that trails have trouble matching. The sight of a white church on a hillside seen from another hillside with a wooded valley between, especially in the fall after the leaves have turned color, is worth the effort to get to the top of the hill. The same with a hilltop view of a river, lake, prairie, or other vista.

SMELLS

The rider will be able to smell a variety of odors as he or she rides through an area. Some of my favorite smells are a freshly-plowed field or newly-mown hay in farm country, lilac bushes, which can be smelled from blocks away if the wind is right, a pine forest (especially after a rainfall), and fallen leaves or, better yet, burning leaves, in the fall. Of course, not all the odors will be pleasant but life isn't perfect--enjoy the good smells and hold your breath past the bad ones.

SOUNDS

Riding through the Black Hills of South Dakota one October my friends and I never saw elk but heard them "bugling" in the distance. It was a cloudy, misty morning and the sound was really eerie. They sounded like the brachiosaurus in the movie "Jurassic Park." On that same trip I was ahead of the others and rounded a curve in the trail at a pretty quick pace, startling a group of deer, a buck and several does, and heard the buck "snort" out a warning to the does, after which they scattered. It was the first time I had heard an actual "buck snort."

The screech of an eagle overhead is impressive and the "gobbling" of wild turkeys, while not as impressive, is enjoyable.

And, of course, the normal sounds, such as the singing of songbirds, especially in spring, when the northern world is coming back to life after a long winter, and the wind in the trees are accentuated by close proximity.

TASTE

The taste and feel of an ice-cold (insert beverage of your choice here) after a long, hot, dry day of bike riding can be wonderful depending on just how long, hot and dry the ride was. Water bottle water will keep you hydrated but is usually warm and not exactly refreshing. And knowing that the long, hot, dry ride is now over makes the ice-cold (insert beverage of your choice here) taste that much better.

Starting to ride bike again may lead you into more and more biking, it may lead to just riding short distances around your neighborhood, or it may lead to hanging the bike in the garage and not using it again. The important thing is to give it a try and give yourself the chance of finding a new form of enjoyment. Riding may not lead to the days and days of enjoyment it has given others, but it may, if you give it a try--all you have to lose is a little time and a little weight. And, who knows, one day, after a pleasant ride (good weather, country scenery, birds chirping, wind in the trees) you may end up saying to yourself, "I can't believe more people don't do this!"

ANECDOTE

In 2004 my friend, Steve, and I were riding The Grand Excursion, an eight-day, 480-mile bike ride from Rock Island, Ill. to St. Paul, Minn. along the Mississippi River. The ride was put on to coincide with the 150-year anniversary celebration of the 1854 event that encouraged western expansion. Numerous riverboats were also making the journey and at each overnight stop several riverboats docked and disgorged their passengers. The town hosting the overnight put on a celebration and, thus, there was a party every night--in each of which we partook heartily.

On the sixth day, we ended up in Red Wing, Minn. after a 65-mile ride, and were hoping for a bit of shuteye before the night's festivities. After getting our tents set up and showers taken, we rolled out our sleeping pads on the ground and stretched out in the warm afternoon sun for a quick nap. Just as we closed our eyes we were shaken by a loud "Boom!" maybe fifty yards from us. It was followed by several more booms, then what sounded like rifle fire--a lot of rifle fire. The booms started up again and lasted for what seemed like a good hour. So much for a nice, quiet nap! We were told there was a group re-enacting a Civil War battle in the field next to the campground. Being somewhat of a history buff I was pretty certain there were no Civil War battles waged anywhere near Minnesota so I was curious. It turns out the battle being re-enacted was the Battle of Gettysburg in which the First Minnesota Regiment had a large, heroic part.

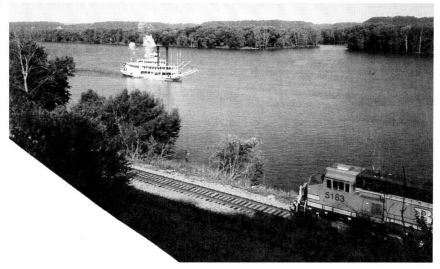

Riverboat on the Mississippi River during The Grand Excursion.

About the Author

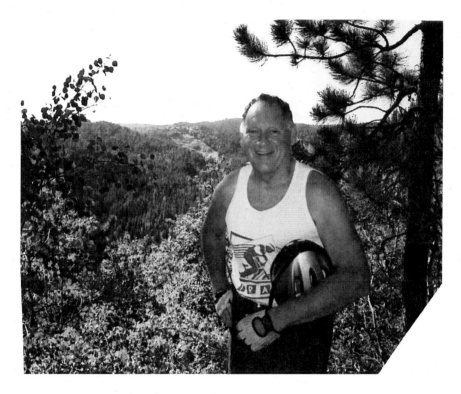

Bruce Wynkoop has been cycling seriously as an adult for twenty-five years. After knee and back pain forced him to give up jogging he needed a form of exercise that wasn't so hard on his body. Starting with short rides and quickly working up to longer ones, he soon came to enjoy it so much that he wondered why more people don't do it. He now averages 2500 miles a season on his road and hybrid bicycles (combined) and has ridden numerous cross-state rides, both in supported rides put on by organizations and self-supported rides with just a couple of friends. He has ridden the Natchez Trace in Mississippi, The Great River Road from St. Paul to St. Louis, the KATY Trail in Missouri, the George Mickelson Trail in South Dakota, around Lake Champlain, through Holland, North Dakota's Theodore Roosevelt National Park and South Dakota's Badlands National Park, and many other interesting places. He considers himself a "serious-casual" cyclist, rides for exercise and pleasure, not for ego, and says, "I don't ride fast, but I can ride all day." He hasn't ridden in the Tour de France, won any cycling awards, or set any records for riding across the country (even for his age group), and has no desire to do so. He has, however, cycled extensively, loves to cycle, and thinks the world would be a better place if more people cycled.